# Contributions to Nephrology

## Vol. 186

Series Editor

Claudio Ronco  Vicenza

# Buttonhole Cannulation

## Current Prospects and Challenges

Volume Editors

Madhukar Misra  Columbia, Mo.

Shigeki Toma  Okinawa

Takahiro Shinzato  Nagoya

23 figures, 3 in color and 9 tables, 2015

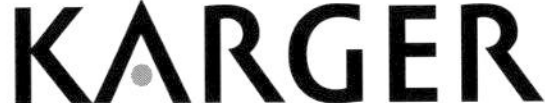

Basel · Freiburg · Paris · London · New York · Chennai · New Delhi ·
Bangkok · Beijing · Shanghai · Tokyo · Kuala Lumpur · Singapore · Sydney

# Contributions to Nephrology

(Founded 1975 by Geoffrey M. Berlyne)

**Madhukar Misra, MD**
Division of Nephrology
University of Missouri Columbia
Columbia, MO 65212 (USA)

**Shigeki Toma, MD**
Toma Clinic
972 Aza-Kochi, Nishihara-cho
Nakagami-gun
Okinawa Prefecture (Japan)

**Takahiro Shinzato, MD**
Daiko Medical Engineering Research
Insititute
4-16-23 Daiko, Higashi-ku
Nagoya-shi, Aichi-ken 461-0043 (Japan)

Library of Congress Cataloging-in-Publication Data

Buttonhole cannulation : current prospects and challenges / volume editors,
Madhukar Misra, Shigeki Toma, Takahiro Shinzato.
     p. ; cm. -- (Contributions to nephrology, ISSN 0302-5144 ; vol. 186)
   Includes bibliographical references and index.
   ISBN 978-3-318-05566-5 (hard cover : alk. paper) -- ISBN 978-3-318-05567-2
(electronic version)
   I. Misra, Madhukar, editor. II. Toma, Shigeki, editor. III. Shinzato,
Takahiro, editor. IV. Series: Contributions to nephrology ; v. 186.
0302-5144
   [DNLM: 1.  Arteriovenous Shunt, Surgical--adverse effects. 2.
Arteriovenous Shunt, Surgical--methods. 3.  Arteriovenous Fistula--therapy.
4.  Infection Control--methods. 5.  Punctures--adverse effects.  W1 CO778UN
v.186 2015 / WG 170]
   RD572
   617.4'61059--dc23
                                                2015022148

Bibliographic Indices. This publication is listed in bibliographic services, including Current Contents® and Index Medicus.



© Copyright 2015 by S. Karger AG, P.O. Box, CH–4009 Basel (Switzerland)
www.karger.com
Printed in Germany on acid-free and non-aging paper (ISO 9706) by Kraft Druck GmbH, Ettlingen
ISSN 0302–5144
e-ISSN 1662–2782
ISBN 978–3–318–05566–5
e-ISBN 978–3–318–05567–2

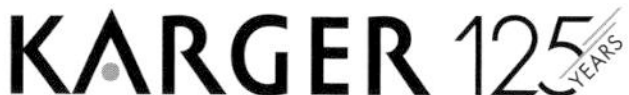

# Contents

Contents

# Preface

Over 40 years have passed since Dr. Zbylut J. Twardowski, a Polish nephrologist, discovered the buttonhole method for the cannulation of the arteriovenous fistula. It was a serendipitous discovery but was soon adopted due to its obvious benefits of decreased puncture pain and extension of the life of the arteriovenous fistula. After about 30 years, this method has recently been the subject of intense scrutiny following reports of higher incidence rates of access-related infections.

Recent research has highlighted the mechanism of buttonhole access-related infections. Interest has also grown in newer techniques related to this method that may have important bearing on the future use of this method. We feel that all such recent research needs to be presented to the scientific community in an easily accessible and readily available format. We hope that this book will foster further scientific inquiry in the medical community about this very important access cannulation technique. Further work in the area of buttonhole-related infections would eventually benefit the patient, without which all research loses its meaning.

In brief, this book is a collection of all relevant information including history, benefits and the latest research related to the buttonhole cannulation method. Despite our best efforts, we could not collect all the relevant work in this field for reasons beyond our control. However, the articles presented in this volume do provide enough material to the reader to achieve two primary objectives: (1) to rekindle an awareness of the advantages of the buttonhole cannulation method and (2) to encourage a critical analysis of possible techniques to overcome current barriers that prevent a wider uptake of this method of cannulation worldwide.

*Madhukar Misra*, Columbia, Mo.
*Shigeki Toma*, Nishihara-cho
*Takahiro Shinzato*, Nagoya

Misra M, Toma S, Shinzato T (eds): Buttonhole Cannulation: Current Prospects and Challenges.
Contrib Nephrol. Basel, Karger, 2015, vol 186, pp 1–12 (DOI: 10.1159/000431159)

# History of the Buttonhole Technique

Madhukar Misra

Division of Nephrology, Department of Medicine, University of Missouri, Columbia, Mo., USA

**Abstract**

The constant side method of access cannulation in hemodialysis, popularly known as the 'buttonhole' method, has an interesting history. Dr. Zbylut J. Twardowski, a Polish nephrologist, discovered this technique by pure serendipity in 1972. A patient with a complicated vascular access history and limited options for cannulation was repeatedly 'stuck' at the same sites by a nurse. Soon it was noticed that the cannulation at the same spot became easier with time. Since the needles were being reused, the sharpness of the needles decreased with time and the bluntness of the needle seemed to minimize the damage to the cannulation tract (another serendipity!). This method soon became popular among patients, and many patients started using this technique. This chapter traces the invention of this technique and its subsequent development following Dr. Twardowski's emigration to the USA.  © 2015 S. Karger AG, Basel

Dr. Twardowski described the discovery of the 'buttonhole' method in his autobiography [1]. From 1969 to 1972, all needle insertions in the Dialysis Center in Bytom, Poland, under his direction were done in different sites of the arterialized vein. In 1971, a 26-year-old lady, Maria Zieleniec-Madejska, was admitted to the center with end-stage renal disease due to chronic glomerulonephritis. She had an arteriovenous fistula created on the left radial artery and cephalic vein, but before it developed she inadvertently hit the anastomosis with a 'Click Clack' – a popular toy at the time. The fistula clotted, but because she needed hemodialysis immediately, she was started, on April 4, 1971, on chronic hemodialysis with an arteriovenous shunt inserted originally into the right femoral artery and femoral vein and later into the left radial artery and the left cephalic vein. In February the following year, an arteriovenous fistula was created on the right radial artery and hemodialysis was started on the fistula in March 1972. The patient had very limited segments suitable for needle insertion. Only one nurse, Sister Helena Kubara was sufficiently experienced to cannulate her fistula. Out of necessity, the insertion of needles was done repeatedly in the same spots. Within a few months the patient noted that needle insertions were not painful and requested not to use lignocaine.

After hearing about the patient's positive experience by word of mouth, other patients requested constant-site needle insertion.

It was observed that the insertion was not painful after the track was created, was accomplished quickly, and that no complications were noted. Eventually this method came to be used in other patients. In the course of 6 months it was accepted by all 16 patients under treatment at that time. After at least a month of Sister Helena performing the technique, other nurses were in a position to cannulate fistulas. The overall results and our experience with the fistulas were published in 1977 [2]. In this paper, seemingly paradoxical observations regarding improvement of fistulas with frequent dialysis up to six times weekly were reported. As can be seen, the discovery of the constant-site method was serendipitous. Dr. Twardowski said that his role was positive in the sense that he did not reject out of hand the discovery made by a patient and a nurse. A report describing specifically the constant-site method of needle insertion was published 2 years later [3]. This paper provided a detailed comparison of different-site versus constant-site needle insertion. A comparison of 4,060 hemodialysis sessions using the different-site method and 6,180 hemodialysis sessions using the constant-site method showed the tremendous advantages of the latter method, particularly with regard to hematoma formations, reinsertions, and patient and nurse preference (table 1). There was a tendency to higher infections at the puncture sites requiring antibiotic treatment, although the difference in comparison to the different-site method was not statistically significant.

For the different-site cannulation method, very sharp needles manufactured by the Seattle Artificial Kidney Supply Co. (Seattle, Wash., USA) were used. Initially the same needles were used for the constant-site method, but they were replaced by needles manufactured by Fabryka Narzędzi Lekarskich i Dentystycznych w Milanówku (Factory of Medical and Dental Instruments in Milanówek, Poland), which were considerably less expensive. These needles were not as sharp as the needles used previously for the different-site method and were reused, which made them even blunter. The bluntness of these needles was advantageous for the constant-site method as they went through the established path without cutting adjacent tissue. New needles were used to establish

**Table 1.** Comparison of the two methods of needle insertion in the original study [3]

|  | Different sites | Constant sites |
| --- | --- | --- |
| Fistulas (n) | 22 | 25 |
| Dialysis session (n) | 4,060 | 6,180 |
| Time for setting up dialysis (min) | 15–25 | 5–15 |
| Reinsertion (%) | 9.91 | 0.96 |
| Hematoma formation (%) | 12.5 | 0.1 |
| Fistula limb failure (n) | 3 | 1 |
| Fistula failure (n) | 1 | 1 |
| Infection requiring ABX (n) | 1 | 3 |
| Patients' preference | no | yes |
| Nurses' preference | no | yes |

ABX = Antibiotics.

the tunnel path and became blunter with reuse, so it was a smooth transition from sharp to blunt needles. It was another serendipitous discovery.

In most patients on thrice-weekly dialysis only two sites were used (fig. 1a). Some patients, however, required more than thrice-weekly dialysis, in which case there were two sites of insertion (fig. 1b, c) that were used alternately as Dr. Twardowski noted 'insertion at the same site day after day is painful' [3]. In 1977 Dr. Twardowski became the Chairman of the Department of Nephrology of the Medical Academy in Lublin and introduced this method where it was used in patients with Cimino-Brescia fistulas and saphenous vein grafts with the same results [3].

The decrease in the rate of hematoma formation was partly contributed to the use of antegrade insertion of the withdrawal (arterial) needle. The original suggestion of the inventors of arteriovenous fistula for hemodialysis was to direct the needle withdrawal retrograde [4]. This practice has been followed by others for many years. One of the reasons was to avoid blood recirculation during hemodialysis; however, blood recirculation does not depend on the needle direction, so there is no good reason for using a retrograde needle direction. Blood recirculation happens when the intended blood flow through the dialyzer is higher than the fistula blood flow, particularly if the needles are inserted very close to each other. In 1973, Woodson and Shapiro [5] from the Division of Thoracic Surgery and Division of Nephrology, Medical College of Ohio (Toledo, Ohio, USA), presented compelling arguments for using an antegrade direction for both needles since a retrograde direction of the withdrawal needle was associated with increased formation of hematomas and pseudoaneurysms. In the original studies on the constant-site method of needle insertion, an antegrade direction for both needles was followed.

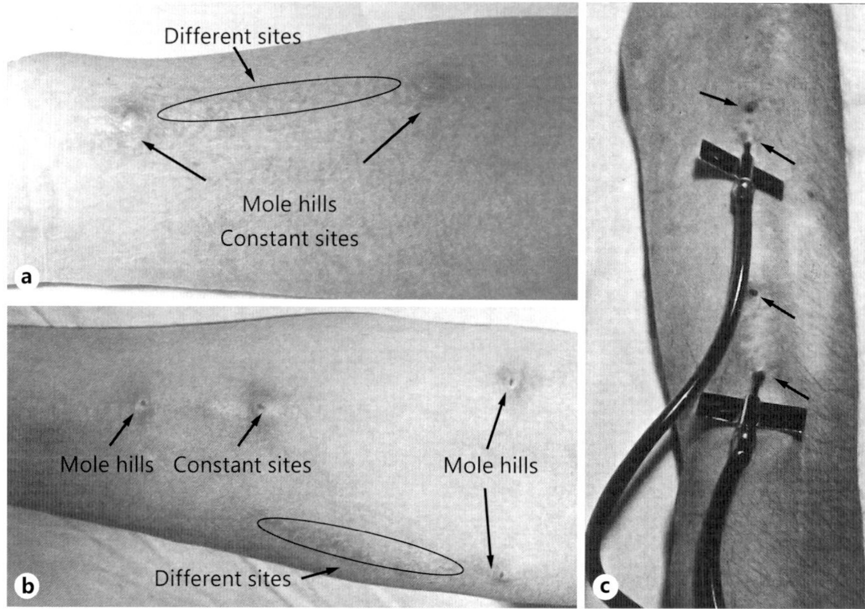


**Fig. 1.** 6-year-old fistula with Polish needles inserted for hemodialysis. There was no oozing from the puncture sites. Note that the hubs are at least 2 mm from the skin and the sites from previous needle insertions are clearly visible (modified from Twardowski and Kubara [3]).

An important factor in arteriovenous fistula use and survival is the blood flow through the dialyzer. Higher blood flow also requires bigger needles (gauge 15 or even 14), which are not favorable for fistula complications. In the original study on constant-site needle insertion, blood flow thorough the dialyzer was always 200 ml/min and needles with outer diameters of 1.6 mm (inner diameter of 1.2 mm, gauge 16) were used [2, 3].

A few years later, Belding Scribner [6, 7] reported his experience with this method in patients with Cimino-Brescia fistulas and confirmed the conclusions of the Twardowski study. In 1984, George Krönung [8] from the University Hospital Bonn (Federal Republic of Germany) presented an analysis of the consequences of repeated fistula punctures and the best technique to avoid fistula damage. Among the three methods (fig. 2), the worst is the area puncture technique, which leads to aneurysms and stenosis. The 'rope-ladder technique' is a better technique in which punctures are evenly distributed along the whole fistula length, and the best technique is the repeated puncture of the same site, which he renamed the 'buttonhole puncture technique'.

After Dr. Twardowski's departure from Bytom, the constant-site method continued to be used for Maria Zieleniec-Madejska, the first patient in whom

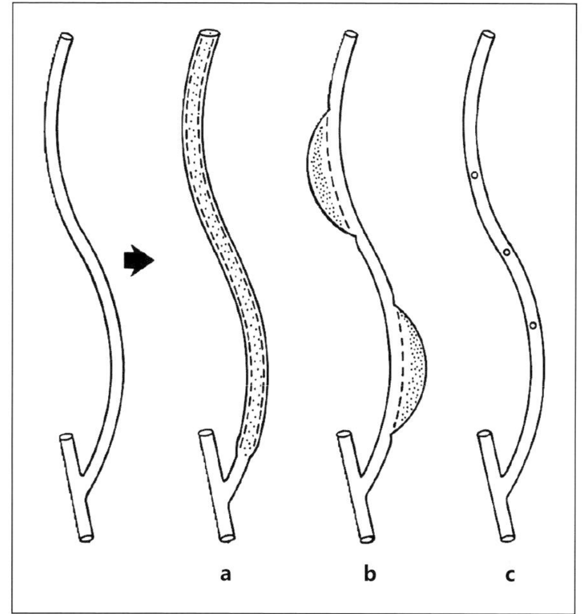

**Fig. 2.** The three types of puncture localization and their morphologic consequences. **a** The rope-ladder method requires a fistula with long segments suitable for cannulations. **b** The area-puncture method, where punctures are done in a confined area, weakens the fistula wall and leads to development of (pseudo) aneurysms and strictures. **c** The buttonhole (constant-site) method is the best and may also be used in fistulas with short segments suitable for sticking [8].



the buttonhole method was attempted. She gradually developed various complications, including arteriosclerosis and dialysis-related amyloidosis. When he was in Kraków in 1993, she visited him to ask for some advice. Given her amyloidosis he suggested transplantation, but her candidacy was ultimately rejected because of very poor arteries. Her fistula was lost in 1998, and it was impossible to create another one, so from 1998 she was dialyzed on intravenous catheters. She developed multiple myeloma and passed away in March 2004 after almost 33 years of hemodialysis. She was probably the longest survivor exclusively on dialysis in Poland at that time.

Dr. Twardowski moved to Columbia (Mo., USA) and joined the faculty in the Division of Nephrology, Department of Medicine, University of Missouri, in 1982. Following the success of the constant-site method of needle insertion in Bytom and Lublin, Dr. Twardowski tried to introduce the method after starting his clinical duties in the Hemodialysis Center at Dialysis Clinic Inc. in 1982. However, there was some skepticism among the nursing staff about the possibility of having a single sticker establish the site, as there was a good deal of staff rotation. Blunt needles were not available, and the nurses reported that the needles did not go through the same needle tunnel but cut the adjacent tissue. As mentioned above, Dr. Twardowski knew that the method was being used in the US by Dr. Scribner and learned that he taught the method to one of his home hemodialysis patients, APL who informed GH, another home hemodialysis patient from Georgia, about the advantages of the method. Both APL and GH only used sharp needles and cannulated themselves. Mr. GH was very interested in new hemodialysis machines; he contacted Rod Kenley, President of Aksys Ltd. and told him about the buttonhole method of needle insertion. In 1994, Rod called Dr. Twardowski and urged him to work on the problem, as it might be important for home hemodialysis programs.

Dr. Twardowski decided to invite GH to the 1st International Symposium on Home Hemodialysis of CAPD (Continuous Ambulatory Peritoneal Dialysis) Conference to present his experience with the method. He also decided to write another paper on the method, as his paper from 15 years earlier was not readily available. In the new paper [9] he presented a history of the method and speculated on why the method had not been popular in spite of excellent initial results. He blamed several factors, including the predominance of graft fistulas in the US that were not tested to determine whether the method was suitable for this kind of access. He also suggested that the currently used needles were too sharp; in Bytom they had serendipitously used blunt needles. Finally, he blamed the organization of the fistula puncture technique on a busy hemodialysis center, the so-called 'multiple sticker' practice. In Bytom, and later in Lublin, only one nurse was initially sufficiently experienced to establish the puncture site. Only after several weeks did other nurses become qualified to cannulate the fistula in the established site. In the majority of centers, stickers were different for each dialysis. The 'single sticker' practice was used for home dialysis, and the results were better as a consequence. In January 1992, along with a change in address, there were also some changes in the hemodialysis nursing staff at Dialysis Clinic Inc. Dr. Twardowski talked again with the nurses and some of them became interested in studying the buttonhole method, but blunter needles were not available.

Aksys Ltd., which was working on the machine for frequent home hemodialysis, had some discussions regarding blood access. One of the top questions that people asked about daily hemodialysis was: 'What about access?' Dr. Twardowski was not particularly concerned, as in the paper he co-authored in 1977 [2] it was noted that frequent dialysis did not deteriorate the fistula – to their surprise, frequent dialysis was even beneficial to the fistula. Dr. Twardowski mentioned in his autobiography that he was a little puzzled that people were concerned about the frequent use of fistulas but not about using high flow dialysis, which had never been proven not to be detrimental to fistulas. As a matter of fact, large needles and high-velocity blood stream from the needle may contribute to the shorter survival of fistulas in the USA compared to Japan and Europe.

Dr. Twardowski contacted William J. Schnell, an engineer at Medisystems Research Corporation (Lakemoor, Ill., USA) and a member of the Board of Directors of Aksys, and they began cooperation in September 1996. Mr. Schnell used electropolishing to prepare several needles with varying degrees of bluntness and asked Dr. Twardowski which one would be appropriate. To remove spikes or burrs, some electropolishing was always done for regular needles, but prolonged electropolishing made the needle blunter. Dr. Twardowski did not have any objective method for measuring bluntness, so he tested them by touching the tip with index finger, not knowing how a particular needle had been prepared. They eventually decided upon two kinds of blunt needles, one with a 45° bevel and the other with a 20° bevel. The nurses established the puncture sites and then started using the blunt needles. Dr. Twardowski first started to work with Mike E. Klusmeyer, RN, Jerry Evans, RN, and Jerry Wells, RN, CNN. After a few months they established that the best needle was the one with the 45° bevel and moderate bluntness. Bill Schnell was notified about the choice, and Medisystems provided the needles for a study. From 1996 to 1998 they studied 16 patients with good results, which were presented by Jerry Wells during the 5th International Symposium on Home Hemodialysis in Charlotte (N.C., USA) in February 1999. This study was done on fistulas. There was a trial of this method on 2 grafts. One patient, who was on home dialysis, was able to use the buttonhole method for 2 months, but he received a transplant so no long-term observation was possible. Another trial was very unsuccessful with no track but multiple holes in a small area of the graft. At that time Dr. Twardowski was so discouraged that he decided not to try it anymore and in his paper said: 'It is also doubtful that the method can be used with conventional PTFE vascular graft fistulas. It would be desirable to test the buttonhole method in the new thicker and stronger grafts such as Diastat or those made of hybrid PTFE' [9].

In 1997 Dr. Twardowski produced a video with GH on the technique of buttonhole needle insertion [10], which was shown for the first time during the 3rd International Symposium on Home Hemodialysis in Denver, Colorado, on February 17, 1997. In this video Mr. GH showed his method of buttonhole cannulation, without any pain, in buttonhole tracks that were several years old. At the same time GH published his experience with the buttonhole method [11]. In this paper Mr. GH, a 16-year home hemodialysis patient, presented the difficulties he had with sticking himself while rotating the sites, including uncertainty whether the selected new site would be appropriate and 'whether I get it or miss it'. In 1990 he met APL who told him about the buttonhole technique, and described his satisfaction with it. APL, who had been on dialysis for almost 20 years, told him that he had three venous and three arterial sites. Mr. GH started using the buttonhole method right away. He also created three arterial and three venous sites, but had to abandon one arterial site. To avoid the risk of infection by puncturing the scab, the risk mentioned in the Krönung paper [8], he removed the scab with sterile forceps and cleaned the site again with povidone-iodine. Mr. GH used the buttonhole technique successfully for over 10 years until he received a successful kidney transplant, and reported from his experience that 'there is no pain with this technique and there is a great sense of confidence in having fixed, well-known sites'.

After some time, Medisystems stopped manufacturing the blunt needles in accordance with Twardowski's request, and began manufacturing very blunt needles that did not require needle guards and were used mostly for subcutaneous catheters, such as Dialock™ (Biolink Corporation, Middleborough, Mass., USA) and LifeSite (VascA, Topsfield, Mass., USA). The needles are called ButtonHole™ Needle Sets with Anti-Stick Dull Bevel. The subcutaneous catheters provided poor results and were ultimately taken off the market. Needles that were too blunt were not suitable for the buttonhole method in many patients. Dr. Twardowski received e-mails and calls from nurses and home patients saying that they could not use the blunt needles as they were too blunt. Out of necessity he advised them to use sharp needles. Dr. Twardowski contacted David Utterberg, the President of Medisystems, to ask him to manufacture needles with intermediate bluntness, so that there would be four types of needles: sharp for the creation of the tunnel, and three kinds of needles with different degrees of bluntness. He suggested grading them by the force needed to puncture the skin (or synthetic material with a resistance similar to skin). David Utterberg promised to work on the problem but encountered some difficulties. Medisystems never returned to making needles of similar dullness to those manufactured by electropolishing in 1996. Dr. Twardowski also asked the same of Tim Dillon of Nipro (US Division), but he was also unable to do it. Nevertheless, Nipro began manufacturing blunt needles, which they called the BioHole™ Needle 'for established access sites only'. These needles are duller than sharp needles but less dull than the Medisystems ButtonHole Needle (fig. 3). JMS North America Corporation (Hayward, Calif., USA) was a third company that made dull needles, which they called Harmony™. Other companies also started making blunt needles, but there is no developed measure to grade their bluntness.

Several centers started to use the buttonhole method with positive results. Patt Peterson, RN, CNN, a Nurse Manager of Professional Services for Medisystems (Seattle, Wash., USA), published a paper in *Nephrology Nursing Journal* describing the method [12].

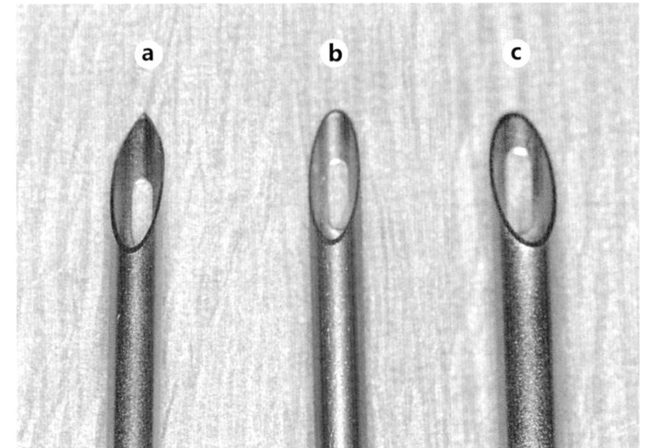

**Fig. 3.** Three kinds of needles: Medisystems Sharp (**a**), Nipro BioHole (**b**), and Medisystems Buttonhole (**c**) (photo by Z. Twardowski).

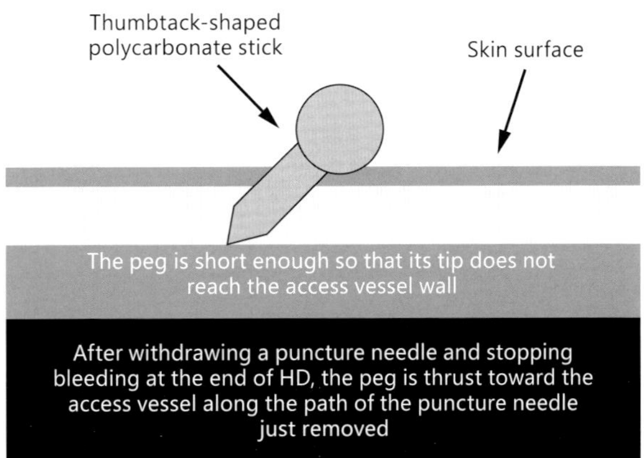


**Fig. 4.** Toma's method of creating a buttonhole tunnel [13].

In Japan, Shigeki Toma, MD, developed a faster method of creating a buttonhole tunnel. Toma et al. [13] explain that after needle removal, 'a dull-tipped, thumbtack-shaped, 5-mm long, polycarbonate peg (BH Stick®, Nipro Corporation, Osaka, Japan), which does not quite reach the access vessel when entering from the skin, is thrust toward the access vessel along the path previously taken by the just-removed dialysis needle' (fig. 4). The tunnel is usually ready after 2 weeks, and a BioHole needle can then be used. Initially the pegs were left in place for 14 days and hemodialysis sessions were performed by puncturing the vessels at sites away from the indwelling peg sites (first-generation time-saving method). This method was used in 55 patients for a total of 18,142 times for up to 25 months. The results were excellent with no serious complications and the authors reported 'the pain of puncture was reduced, if not completely eliminated'. In the second-generation method the punctures for consecutive dialyses were done with blunt needles through the track already formed by the peg left in place after removal of the peg. These steps were repeated at each hemodialysis session for 14 days. The results with the second-generation method in 37 patients were also excellent with diminished or eliminated pain. Only 1 patient had enough erythema to suggest possible infection.

Robert M. Lindsay and his colleagues [14] from the Optimal Dialysis Research Unit, London Health Sciences Centre (London, Ont., Canada) were treating 11 patients with daily hemodialysis and 12 with nocturnal hemodialysis. More than 80% of the patients on daily or nocturnal hemodialysis elected to use the buttonhole technique and successfully performed dialysis sessions for 18 months. Robert S. Lockridge Jr. [15] and his colleagues from Lynchburgh (Va., USA) introduced a nocturnal home hemodialysis program in 1997. Patients with arteriovenous fistulas were trained to cannulate their access with 16-gauge needles using the buttonhole method. Two venous and two arterial buttonholes were established. The same nurse performed cannulation until the patient was able to perform the procedure. The method was successfully used for many years. Lynda Ball [16], BS, BSN, RN, CNN, the Quality Improvement Coordinator of the Northwest Renal Network (Seattle, Wash., USA) reported her initial positive experience with the buttonhole technique in 2005.

Rosa M. Marticorena and her colleagues from the Division of Nephrology, St. Michael Hospital, University of Toronto (Toronto, Ont., Canada) presented their experience with the buttonhole method in a busy full-care hemodialysis unit. To secure proper development of buttonhole track, only 1–3 experienced cannulators per patient used sharp needles. After the track was created and cannulations were easily achieved with dull needles, additional cannulators were incorporated with guidance from a mentor. The authors found that pain decreased the longer the track was used. In addition, hemostasis time after dialysis decreased from 24 to 15 min [17]. In 2005, the Japanese Society for Dialysis Therapy published guidelines for vascular access [18]. They recommended to use buttonhole puncturing in patients who complain of intense pain. They also stated that 'a fixed puncture route for buttonhole method is created by removing the puncture needle after routine dialysis and placing a short post that only reaches near the surface of the arterialized vein in the same puncture route for 14 days'.

Lynda Ball [19] published an excellent description of the creation of the buttonhole track, removal of scab, and careful use of antimicrobial agent or solution at the Northwest Kidney Center in Seattle where many quotidian dialysis patients were being treated. She stated that 'it has been found that the buttonhole technique is a viable technique for reducing pain of cannulation and may help those patients who have needle fears. And, finally, the buttonhole technique can promote self-cannulation and allow patients to be self-sufficient, more confident, and in control of the biggest aspect of their treatment – the access'.

There has also been a report from Ball et al. [20] of a multicenter experience with buttonhole in the Pacific Northwest. According to this study, 'the patients have reported very high satisfaction with this technique, with both a reduction of complications and pain associated with cannulation'. In her e-mail to Dr. Twardowski in August 2007, she remarked that 'buttonhole has caught on like wildfire'.

The buttonhole technique continues to evolve. There have been concerns related to increased incidence of infection. Obviously, further studies are needed to develop the best possible technique of cannulation and the best tools for this method, a detailed description of which is beyond the scope of this chapter.

## References


1 Twardowski ZJ: Around the world with nephrology: an autobiography. Singapore, World Scientific Publishing, 2013, pp 171–173 and 242–248.

2 Twardowski Z, Lebek R, Kubara H: Six-year clinical experience with the creation and use of internal arteriovenous fistulas in patients treated with repeated haemodialysis (in Polish). Pol Arch Med Wewn 1977;57:205–214.

3 Twardowski Z, Kubara H: Different sites versus constant sites of needle insertion into arteriovenous fistulas for treatment by repeated dialysis. Dial Transplant 1979;8:978–979.

4 Brescia MJ, Cimino JE, Appel K, Hurwich BJ: Chronic hemodialysis using venipuncture and a surgically created arteriovenous fistula. N Engl J Med 1966;275:1089–1092.

5 Woodson RD, Shapiro RS: Antegrade vs retrograde cannulation for percutaneous hemodialysis. Dial Transplant 1974;3:29–30.

6 Scribner BH: Circulatory access – still a major concern. Proc Eur Dial Transplant Assoc 1983;19:95–98.

7 Scribner BH: The overriding importance of vascular access. Dial Transplant 1984;13:625.

8 Krönung G: Plastic deformation of Cimino fistula by repeated puncture. Dial Transplant 1984;13:635–638.

9 Twardowski ZJ: Constant site (buttonhole) method of needle insertion for hemodialysis. Dial Transplant 1995;24:559–560, 576.

10 Twardowski ZJ, Harper G: Buttonhole Method of Needle Insertion into Arteriovenous Fistulas (video). Columbia, Academic Support Center, University of Missouri, 1997.

11 Harper G: The buttonhole technique of fistula access: a personal experience. Home Hemodial Int 1997;1:41–42.

12 Peterson P: Fistula cannulation: the buttonhole technique. Nephrol Nurs J 2002;29:195.

13 Toma S, Shinzato T, Fukui H, Nakai S, Miwa M, takai I, Maeda K: A timesaving method to create a fixed puncture route for the buttonhole technique. Nephrol Dial Transplant 2003;18:2118–2121.

14 Lindsay RM, Leitch R, Heidenheim AP, Kortas C: The London daily/nocturnal hemodialysis study – study design, morbidity, and mortality results. Am J Kidney Dis 2003; 42(1 suppl):S5–S12.

15 Pipkin M, Craft V, Spencer M, Lockridge RS Jr: Six years of experience with nightly home hemodialysis. Hemodial Int 2004;8:349–353.

16 Ball LK: Improving arteriovenous fistula cannulation skills. Nephrol Nurs J 2005;32:611–617.

17 Marticorena RM, Hunter J, Macleod S, Petershofer E, Dacouris N, Donelly S, Goldstein MB: The salvage of aneurysmal fistulae utilizing a modified buttonhole cannulation technique and multiple cannulators. Hemodial Int 2006;10:193–200.

18 Ohira S, Naito H, Amano I, Azuma N, Ikeda K, Kukita K, Goto Y, Sakai S, Shinzato T, Sugimoto T, Takemoto Y, Haruguchi H, Hino I, Hiranaka T, Mizuguchi J, Miyata A, Murotani N; Japanese Society for Dialysis Therapy: 2005 Japanese Society for Dialysis Therapy guidelines for vascular access construction and repair for chronic hemodialysis. Ther Apher Dial 2006;10:449–462.

19 Ball LK: The buttonhole technique for arteriovenous fistula cannulation. Nephrol Nurs J 2006;33:299–304.

20 Ball LK, Treat L, Riffle V, Scherting D, Swift L: A multi-center perspective of the buttonhole technique in the Pacific Northwest. Nephrol Nurs J 2007;34:234–241.

Madhukar Misra, Professor of Medicine
Division of Nephrology, Department of Medicine, University of Missouri Columbia
C420 CSE Building, 5 Hospital Drive
Columbia, MO 65212 (USA)
E-Mail misram@health.missouri.edu

Misra M, Toma S, Shinzato T (eds): Buttonhole Cannulation: Current Prospects and Challenges.
Contrib Nephrol. Basel, Karger, 2015, vol 186, pp 13–20 (DOI: 10.1159/000431160)

# The Impact of Buttonhole Cannulation on Patients and Staff in Hemodialysis Facilities

Tomonari Ogawa[a] · Etsuko Harada[b] · Yuki Kanayama[c] ·
Atsuko Tanabe[b] · Megumi Inamura[a] · Tota Kiba[a] ·
Taisuke Shimizu[a] · Takatsugu Iwashita[a] · Yosuke Tayama[a] ·
Akihiko Matsuda[a] · Hajime Hasegawa[a]

[a]Department of Nephrology and Blood Purification, [b]Division of Nursing, and [c]Division of Medical
Engineer Service, Saitama Medical Center, Saitama Medical University, Saitama, Japan

## Abstract

The two reasons that patients desire buttonhole cannulation are avoidance of puncture
pain and extension of arteriovenous fistula life. Despite the desire to receive buttonhole
cannulation by many patients, medical staff at most local hemodialysis facilities tend to
hesitate to implement the cannulation method. This method is used on patients in the
dialysis unit at Saitama Medical Center, but tends to be discontinued for those patients
upon their transfer to local hemodialysis facilities. Medical staff members of one local hemodialysis facility report the percentage of patients on the buttonhole method was 53%
in 2007, but that it sharply decreased to 17% in 2013. Hesitation by local hemodialysis
facilities to adopt the buttonhole method is due to, but not limited to, several factors.
These factors include the frequently occurring trampoline effect, the difficulty of removing scabs, formation of a false buttonhole track, and the pain from insertion of a dull needle. Perceived differences in the value of buttonhole cannulation may potentially affect
communication between patients and staff in local hemodialysis facilities.

© 2015 S. Karger AG, Basel

The number of chronic dialysis patients in Japan is over 300,000 [1]. Most of
these patients select in-center hemodialysis over peritoneal dialysis and kidney
transplants [1]. A small number of patients on hemodialysis, however, do switch

their treatment modality to peritoneal dialysis. The main reason for the switch may be vascular access trouble, including pain due to cannulation of an arterio-venous fistula (AVF) with sharp needles.

The skill of each in-charge staff member in a dialysis center may vary, which potentially results in differences in the severity of puncture pain felt by the patient. Therefore, dialysis center staff tend to experience mental stress when they attempt to puncture the AVF of a patient. Such mental stress could induce errors during the cannulation. Such mental stress is expected to decrease when buttonhole cannulation is implemented; however, introduction of this method is occasionally observed as having a negative impact on communication between patients and staff in local hemodialysis facilities. Thus, in this article, we describe the psychological influence of the buttonhole method on both patients and medical staff in local hemodialysis facilities.

## Rope-Ladder Cannulation and Buttonhole Cannulation

The rope-ladder method, a cannulation method using sharp needles, has been the most common approach for cannulation of AVF to date. While using the rope-ladder method, dialysis center staff are often tense and use extreme care to prevent any errors during cannulation. Punctures of the AVF in the narrow range during every hemodialysis session cause the development of stenosis in the AVF. The vessel is accordingly punctured in as wide a range as possible. Consequently, sites that are difficult to cannulate may lead to stress in the medical staff in hemodialysis facilities.

A buttonhole cannulation, developed by Twardowski, may be an effective approach to prevent potential error during cannulation. Twardowski and Kubara [2] called this unique method the 'constant-site puncture method'. This method was renamed the 'buttonhole puncture technique' by Krönung [3]. In this article, this method is referred to as the 'buttonhole method'.

Training and experience are necessary to acquire skills for the buttonhole method. In particular, extensive time is necessary to acquire skills for creating a buttonhole track and for inserting a dull needle that reaches the AVF wall into the AVF lumen through the buttonhole flap. Regarding a buttonhole track, Toma et al. [4] devised an easy method to create the buttonhole track by indwelling a small stick in the sharp needle track. On the other hand, readily inserting a dull needle into the AVF lumen through the flap is difficult. In other words, perhaps limited to Japan, a trampoline effect occurs too frequently. Therefore, more time is required for readily inserting a dull needle into the AVF lumen in Japan.



Ogawa et al.

## Introduction of Buttonhole Method in Local Hemodialysis Facilities

In our dialysis unit at Saitama Medical Center, we have been proactively introducing buttonhole cannulation. However, in most local hemodialysis facilities in the area surrounding the Saitama Medical Center, medical staff tend to hesitate to implement the buttonhole method.

We frequently learn of buttonhole cannulation being discontinued at a local hemodialysis facility upon a patient being moved there from our facility where the patient had been receiving cannulation by this method. The main reason for discontinuation of buttonhole cannulation in the local facility is lack of experience of the staff in performing buttonhole cannulation in addition to lack of skill.

To solve this problem, we gave lectures to medical staff in local hemodialysis facilities in the area surrounding Saitama Medical Center for the purpose of allowing them to perform various buttonhole cannulation techniques. These lectures have successfully led to a gradual increase in facilities willing to introduce buttonhole cannulation.

## Patients' View of Buttonhole Cannulation

During the period from December 2005 to May 2006, we interviewed 57 patients on the buttonhole method and 63 patients on the rope-ladder method. This inquiry was conducted with regard to cannulation of AVF for both methods.

### Interview of Patients Concerning the Buttonhole Method

Patients decided to receive the buttonhole method on the advice of doctors or nurses, or based on their own will. Among patients who chose the buttonhole method, according to interview results, 38% of the patients chose buttonhole cannulation expecting alleviation of puncture pain, 18% expecting extension of AVF life, and 12% expecting prevention of false cannulation (fig. 1).

After the start of buttonhole cannulation, 35% of the patients reported that pain due to needle insertion was alleviated, whereas 19% of the patients mentioned that the pain was not alleviated. Another 14% of the patients reported that their fear of punctures was reduced after buttonhole cannulation was performed. According to the same interview, 22% of the patients reported that they had pain when a scab created at the entry site was removed, and approximately 21% complained that the buttonhole method required more time for cannulation (table 1).

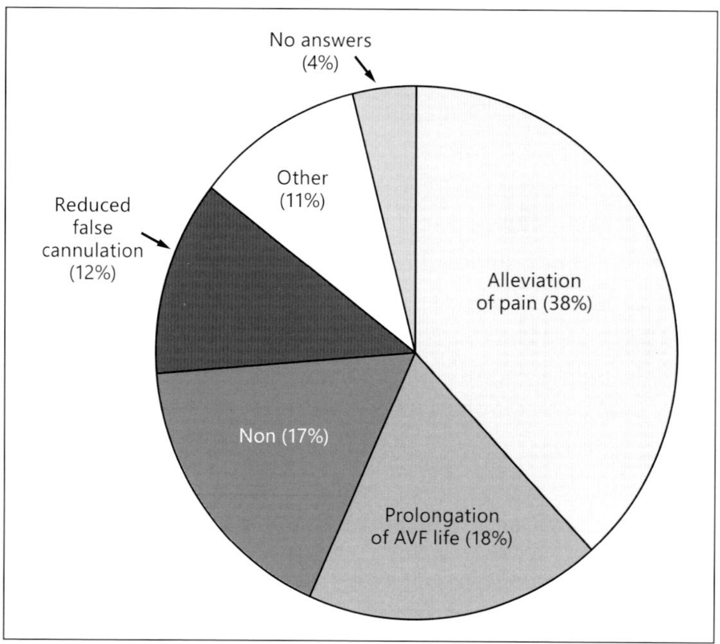


**Fig. 1.** Buttonhole method outcomes (n = 57).

**Table 1.** Outcomes after the start of buttonhole cannulation (n = 57)

| Advantages | Disadvantages |
| --- | --- |
| Alleviation of pain according to 20 patients (35%) | No alleviated of pain according to 11 patients (19%) |
| Shortened time needed for hemostasis according to 9 patients (6%) | Prolonged time needed for hemostasis according to 3 patients (5%) |
| Lessened fear of punctures according to 4 patients (7%) | Pain at the time of scab removal according to 13 patients (23%) |
| Procedure more comfortable according to 4 patients (7%) | Longer cannulation time according to 12 patients (21%) |

Moreover, 84% of the patients reported that they wanted to continue buttonhole cannulation. Thus, most patients wanted to continue buttonhole cannulation once they experienced the method, irrespective of motivation for introduction of the buttonhole method, any advice from doctors or nurses, or their own volition.



Ogawa et al.

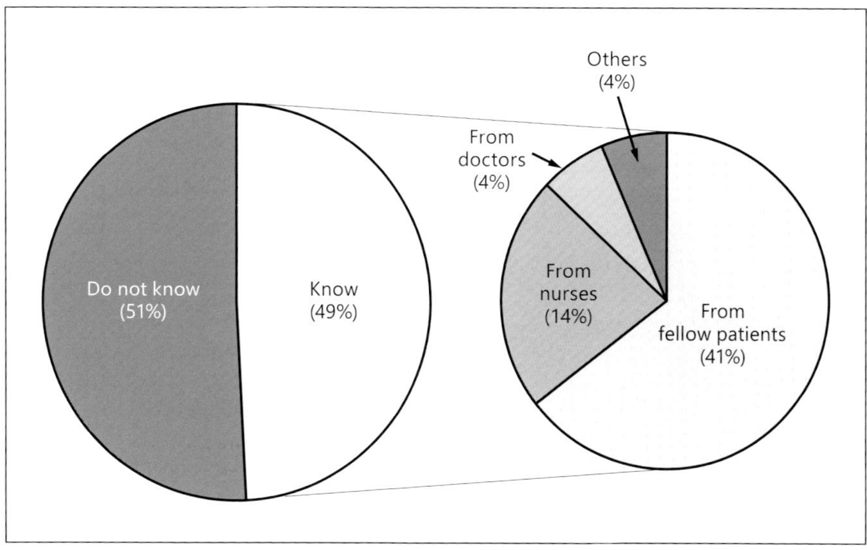


**Fig. 2.** Results of the patient interviews concerning the rope-ladder method (n = 63).

*Interview of Patients Concerning the Rope-Ladder Method*

As shown in figure 2, 32 (51%) of 63 patients interviewed were not aware of the buttonhole method, whereas 31 (49%) patients were. Twenty (65%) of the 31 patients who knew of the buttonhole method had received information regarding the method from fellow patients. Of the 32 patients who were not aware of the buttonhole method, 13 (41%) wished to change their cannulation from the rope-ladder method to the buttonhole method after they learned about buttonhole cannulation from medical staff.

The reasons for the desire to change treatment modality were alleviation of the puncture pain, prolongation of AVF life, and reduction of false cannulation. Among the 13 patients who changed cannulation method from the rope-ladder method to the buttonhole method in response to advice from medical staff, 5 patients reported alleviation of pain after the start of the buttonhole cannulation, whereas 2 patients reported that their pain had not been relieved.

After changing the cannulation method, false cannulation was reduced in 3 of the above 13 patients, and fear of cannulation was reduced in 2 patients. All of these 13 patients complained of pain at the time of scab removal. Out of these 13 patients, 7 patients wanted to continue buttonhole cannulation, but 6 patients were not certain whether they wanted to continue this method.

**Staff Acceptance of the Buttonhole Method in Local Facilities**

Despite a positive reception among many patients who have received buttonhole cannulation, most local hemodialysis facilities remain hesitant to introduce this method. According to the medical staff at one local facility, the percentage of patients on buttonhole cannulation was 53% in their facility in 2007, but the ratio decreased to 17% in 2013.

According to a survey questionnaire of 129 medical professionals involved in providing hemodialysis over 10.7 ± 7.0 years, 103 (80%) abandoned buttonhole cannulation due to several factors, including the frequent incidence of the trampoline effect, the burden of scab removal, and longer time required for cannulation.


**Discussion**

Patients feel a variety of stress factors when they receive hemodialysis [5]. Puncture pain may be a prominent form of stress. Severity of puncture pain may be dependent on factors for patients and puncture skill of medical staff. Therefore, some patients blame poor skill of the medical staff for the severity of the pain they experience, whereas factors acknowledged by medical staff are usually those relating to the patients. Thus, communication errors can occasionally occur between patients and medical staff.

In order to solve such potential friction between patients and medical staff, the cannulation method with less puncture pain is desired. Thus, high expectation for the buttonhole cannulation emerges from some patients as a less painful cannulation method. Nevertheless, local hemodialysis facilities unfortunately hesitate to introduce the buttonhole cannulation method. As mentioned above, for example, the percentage of the patients on buttonhole cannulation decreased from 53% in 2007 to 17% in 2013 in one local hemodialysis facility.

In many local hemodialysis facilities, medical staff have apparently been avoiding the use of buttonhole cannulation, although they understand that the patients are ready to be cannulated by the buttonhole method. This is a complicated situation as outlined by the survey. According to this survey, buttonhole cannulation is favorable for patients because of less puncture pain. However, the method is unfavorable for medical staff because of the frequent occurrence of the trampoline effect and a longer puncture procedure, which includes scab removal. When buttonhole cannulation is not smoothly performed, medical staff, who are under time constraints, are often forced to avoid its use primarily owing to longer time required for puncture.

As summarized in table 2, there are differences in values between the patients and medical staff. Although buttonhole cannulation has been introduced to

**Table 2.** Differences in value between patients and medical staff

| Problems | Patient side | Medical staff side |
| --- | --- | --- |
| Scab removal | Scab must be removed to prevent infection, but the procedure is painful | Scab removal is a time-consuming procedure |
| Technique | Medical staff need to improve their cannulation skill | Successful BH needling is quite difficult |
| Time | Lack of skill by medical staff results in more time required to perform BH cannulation | Successful BH cannulation inherently requires more time |
| | Further training required | BH cannulation is a time-consuming procedure |

BH = Buttonhole cannulation.

lessen the burden of the patients, the procedure has negatively impacted communication between patients and medical staff in some cases.

If medical staff improve their buttonhole cannulation skills and the method for scab removal is revised to make it easier, the buttonhole method will prevail across Japan. Recently, Toma et al. [6] reported that they solved the problem of the trampoline effect by creating a buttonhole track by repeated punctures of the fistular vessel with sharp needles as performed in other countries besides Japan. Moreover, Shinzato et al. [7] succeeded in removing scabs in advance before patients visited their hemodialysis facilities for the next hemodialysis session. They applied a wound moist-healing method to the entry site after hemodialysis and then, during bathing, wiped off the created scab. If these novel techniques are applied in local hemodialysis facilities, all of the problems mentioned above would be solved and the buttonhole method would prevail even in Japan.

## Conclusion

The buttonhole method is beneficial for patients because of reduced puncture pain, whereas it is stressful for staff in local hemodialysis facilities because of a longer puncture procedure, including scab removal.

## Acknowledgments

Thanks to the medical staff of Blood Purification Division of Saitama Medical Center, and Dr. Hirohisa Yamamoto, Akemi Tanabe, the chief nurse, and the medical staff of Kawagoe Ekimae Clinic Ishikawa Kinenkai Medical Group for completing this thesis.

## Disclosure Statment

This thesis is the revision of my presentation at the 52nd annual meeting of The Japanese Society of Dialysis Therapy – (June 2007 in Osaka). This thesis includes the content approved by The Ethics Committee of Saitama Medical Center, Saitama Medical University. The authors have no conflicts of interest to report.

## References


1 Nakai S, Watanabe Y, Masakane I, et al: Overview of regular dialysis treatment in Japan (as of 31 December 2011). Ther Apher Dial Dec 2013;17:567–611.

2 Twardowski Z, Kubara H: Different sites versus constant sites of needle insertion into arteriovenous fistulas for treatment by repeated dialysis. Dial Transplant 1979;8:978–980.

3 Krönung G: Plastic deformation of Cimino fistula by repeated puncture. Dial Transplant 1984;13:635–638.

4 Toma S, Shinzato T, Fukui H, et al: A time-saving method to create a fixed puncture route for the buttonhole technique. Nephrol Dial Transplant 2003;18:2118–2121.

5 Kohli S, Batra P, Aggarwal HK: Anxiety, locus of control, and coping strategies among end-stage renal disease patients undergoing maintenance hemodialysis. Indian J Nephrol 2011;21:177–181.

6 Toma S: New method to prevent trampoline effect (abstract). 7th Congr Int Soc Hemodial, Ginowan City, 2014, p 60.

7 Shinzato T, Shibata K, Fukui H, et al: New treatment method for the buttonhole entry site that leads to formation of no scab or a very small scab (abstract). 7th Congr Int Soc Hemodial, Ginowan City, 2014, p 63.



Tomonari Ogawa
Department of Nephrology and Blood Purification
Saitama Medical Center, Saitama Medical University
1981 Kamoda, Kawagoe-shi
Saitama 350-8550 (Japan)
E-Mail togawa@saitama-med.ac.jp

Misra M, Toma S, Shinzato T (eds): Buttonhole Cannulation: Current Prospects and Challenges.
Contrib Nephrol. Basel, Karger, 2015, vol 186, pp 21–32 (DOI: 10.1159/000431165)

# Buttonhole Tunnel Tract Creation with the BioHole® Buttonhole Device

Jennie King

Renal Department, Royal Berkshire Hospital, Reading, UK

## Abstract

***Background:*** Cannulation, and in particular, skilled cannulation is the cornerstone to preserving the arteriovenous fistula, the lifeline for a patient receiving long-term hemodialysis therapy. The buttonhole cannulation method has seen a huge revival in the 2000s, but it can sometimes prove challenging to implement successfully. This chapter discusses and describes the method of creating a buttonhole tract using the BioHole® device (a sterile polycarbonate peg), and describes the associated advantages and disadvantages. In a busy hemodialysis unit, use of the thumbtack-shaped 5-mm peg allows a fixed puncture route to be created quickly in just 7–14 days. The peg is placed at the site where the sharp puncture needle has just been removed by the designated primary cannulator. The peg remains in place until the next dialysis session when it is removed, the dialysis therapy completed as usual, and a new peg is inserted after hemostasis has been achieved. These steps are repeated for 1–2 weeks. Once the tunnel is formed, use of the peg is no longer needed and a blunt-ended puncture needle is inserted along the track each time. Buttonhole cannulation using the BioHole peg device offers advantages including reduced risk of needling complications and arteriovenous fistula failure, speedy transition to blunt needles, the tunnel track remaining narrow thus reducing the risk of developing an exit site infection, and suitability in difficult sites. Possible disadvantages are increased cost for purchase of the pegs during the track break-in period and potential complications such as discomfort, bleeding, and risk of infection. These risks/disadvantages minimize after the transition to blunt needles which in itself is a safer option than using sharp needles. As supported by KDOQI (2006) and the UK Renal Association (2011), adoption of the buttonhole method as the cannulation technique of choice is recommended in the majority of patients undergoing hemodialysis who have a native fistula. 

**Table 1.** KDOQI and UK Renal Association guidelines

| |
|---|
| NKF KDOQI guidelines, 2006<br>II 3.3 Buttonhole:<br>'Patients with fistula access should be considered for buttonhole (constant-site) cannulation' |
| UK Renal Association: Vascular<br>Access for Haemodialysis 2011<br>Guideline 4.2 – Needling technique<br>'We suggest that buttonhole is the preferred needling technique (2B)' |

Skilled cannulation is the cornerstone to preserving the arteriovenous fistula (AVF), the lifeline for a patient receiving long-term hemodialysis (HD) therapy. In recent years, the method of cannulating the AVF has been closely scrutinized with several published clinical trials and case reports linking the impact of cannulation technique on AVF and graft survival. Cannulation using the buttonhole (BH) method is suggested in KDOQI (2006) [1] and UK Renal Association (2011) [2] guidelines for vascular access (table 1), and the method has enjoyed a huge revival globally in the 2000s. However, it can pose challenges to implement successfully and devices especially designed for this purpose can be helpful. This chapter discusses and describes the method of creating a BH tract using the BioHole® BH device also known as the BioHole stick device (a tiny sterile polycarbonate peg), and describes the associated advantages and disadvantages.

## Background

The BH technique was first described by Twardowski and Kubara [3] in the mid-1970s and was developed to help patients with limited puncture sites. Due to the restricted number of hospital-based HD units at the time, many patients were performing their own HD at home and this technique was found to be ideal for self-needling where fistula needles are inserted into exactly the same puncture site for each dialysis treatment. The BH method can create confidence and reliability for a self-needling patient. However, the requirement for the exact same puncture site cannulation has been one of the biggest barriers to the acceptance of the BH technique [4]. As hospital and satellite-based HD services developed strongly during the 1980s in the UK, and with the advent of peritoneal dialysis, the BH method and home HD treatment faded.

**Table 2.** Advantages and disadvantages when using a BioHole peg

| |
| --- |
| *Advantages* |
| Simple to use – for staff and patients |
| Transition to blunt needles quickly – within 7–21 days |
| Useful for developing BH in difficult sites |
| Keeps tunnel track narrow |
| Less needling complications |
| *Disadvantages* |
| Requirement to keep peg covered/clean/dry while in situ |
| Extra cost |
| Peg can be uncomfortable or cause bleeding |
| Small risk of local infection |

## Factors Required for Successful Buttonhole Cannulation

As the BH technique is a cannulation method where the AVF is cannulated in the exact same spot using the same angle and same depth each time, it has been strongly recommended that the same person (primary cannulator) undertake the cannulation process until the tunnel track of scar tissue is formed so as to minimize the risk of creating false tracks or enlarging the tunnel while in the formation stage. Using sharp needles, it may take anywhere from 7 days to 12 weeks for scar tissue (from the repeated same site cannulation) to form the tunnel track. Other researchers report a median of 11 sharp needles (range: 5–44) are required to create a mature track [5, 6]. Repeated and prolonged use of sharp needles in the tunnel track is thought to cut and damage the track and possibly lead to vascular access complications [7]. It is recommended that once the tunnel track is established, other competent staff can then cannulate with blunt needles [4], which is now considered a safer option due to the risk of needle stick injury to staff and patients with sharp needles. Table 2 provides a full list of associated advantages and disadvantages.

Staff working patterns in busy dialysis units that operate, for instance, on a 6-day schedule pose logistical problems, so it is unlikely that the same person is with the patient on a regular basis. However, with the development of the sterile BioHole polycarbonate peg, a fixed puncture route can be established in a much shorter period of time (1–2 weeks), making the BH technique a more feasible and effective option [8–10]. The successful establishment of the BH technique in a busy HD unit using multiple cannulators has been shown to be possible [11]. Published literature from an early German study reported their patients using the BH method for home HD not only reported favorable results for potential needling complications, but also listed fistula 5-year survival rates (from initial

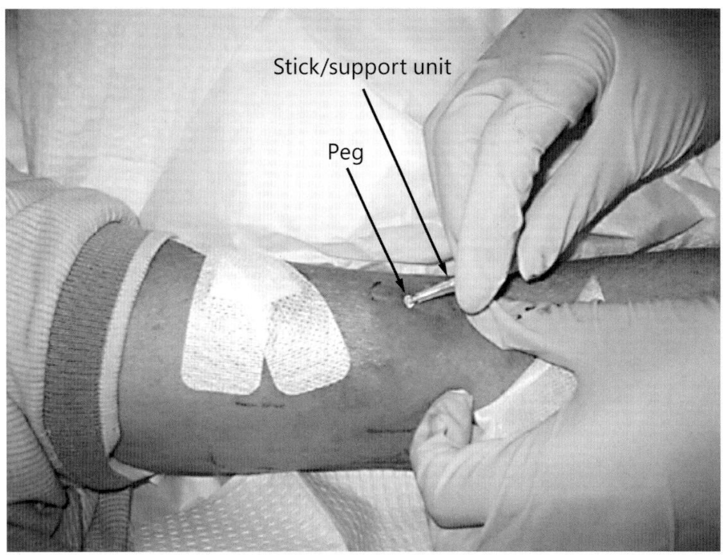


**Fig. 1.** Peg insertion.

cannulation) as 97.4% in their home patients and 87% in their outpatients [12]. Similar results were seen for in-center patients in recent research conducted in the UK [13] where fistula survival at 1 year was significantly increased for patients using the BH method (100%) when compared with rotating-sites cannulation using sharp needles (86%). A case study of more than 7,000 patients investigated the impact of cannulation technique on fistula and graft survival and detected an association, recommending the organization of a large-scale clinical trial to facilitate clinical, evidence-based practice guidelines [14].

## Use of a Polycarbonate Peg

In a busy HD unit, the use of the thumbtack-shaped 5-mm polycarbonate peg allows a fixed puncture route to be created quickly in just 7–14 days, which is a major benefit. The peg is placed at the site where the sharp puncture needle has just been removed by the designated primary cannulator. The peg remains in place until the next dialysis session when it is removed and the dialysis therapy completed as usual; afterwards, a new peg is inserted after hemostasis has been achieved. These steps are repeated for 1–2 weeks. Once the tunnel is formed, use of the peg is no longer necessary and a blunt-ended puncture needle is inserted along the track each time. Figures 1 and 2 show the components of the BioHole stick – the diamond shaped peg that sits at the entrance to the tunnel and the

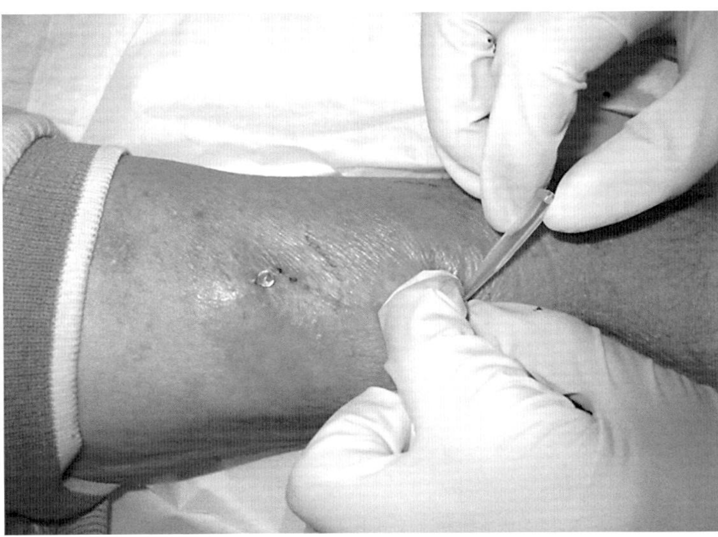

**Fig. 2.** Peg insertion.

stick/support unit device used to position it towards the tunnel. Figure 1 shows the peg being inserted via the introducer, which is twisted off leaving the diamond-head protruding. It is important to note that the peg is tiny and only sits in part of the tunnel and not in the blood vessel. Occasionally, in a very shallow new fistula, it may be difficult to position the peg and bleeding is sometimes caused while the peg is being inserted. If this happens, the peg is removed and the process is tried again next time.

BioHole BH devices (pegs) are marketed in a sterile pack with two devices in each box. They are for single-use only. Guidelines should be followed closely – pegs are inserted after dialysis into sharp needle tracks and generally needed for the first 6 dialysis sessions. Strict aseptic technique must be adopted during peg insertion as there is an increased risk of local infection while the pegs are being used, as the skin integrity is broken. A steady hand wearing new sterile gloves inserts the peg by holding the 'support unit'. Once the peg is in place, the support unit is twisted off and discarded. Sterile forceps could be used instead. The peg sits in the tunnel between the skin and tissue – it should not penetrate into the fistula vein. The peg works in a similar way to an ear ring piercing, with scar tissue forming around the peg while it is in situ on the nondialysis days. To prevent peg dislodgement and maintain skin integrity, it is recommended that the pegs, once in situ, are covered with hypoallergenic plasters which may prevent plaster sensitivity to skin (as the plaster must remain covering the peg until the next dialysis session). During this short period, it is important to remind the patient to take extra care to keep the pegs covered, clean, and dry, and discourage activities such as direct bathing over the site, hard physical labor/exercise, etc. Occasionally at home, patients have experienced discomfort or bleeding while using the peg. As a precaution, in case this should happen, teach the patient how to remove the peg using a clean technique (patient must wash his/her hands thoroughly with soap and warm water, and dry them using a clean towel) and to cover the site immediately with a plaster.

## Evidence for Using the BioHole Device

In 2008, after receiving training and guidance from colleagues in Belgium who were using the BioHole peg, a UK dialysis team researched the effect of BH cannulation using the polycarbonate peg on in-center HD fistula outcomes and needling complications with favorable results [13]. In this randomized controlled trial, the control group (70 patients) continued to dialyze using 15-gauge sharp needles (length: 25 mm), using the practice with which all dialysis nurses were already familiar and competent to perform. In the intervention group (70 patients), the BH method (a new technique for all staff) was initially only performed by the HD ward manager who was subsequently responsible for training her colleagues. BH track formation was allocated to competent staff (primary cannulator) who agreed to follow the BH clinical guidance and could follow the patients' shift allocation for the next 6–8 dialysis sessions. The track former or primary cannulator was sometimes supported by a buddy (who had to be present during early BH cannulation) although the aim was to have only one cannulator perform the sharp needling and peg placement during the tunnel track formation. Initial guidance was to use sharp needles and the peg 6 times (i.e. for 2 weeks) and then attempt the transition to blunt needles. The track former selected the BH site, sometimes with guidance from the vascular access nurse and SonaSite ultrasound machine. Ideally, a straight length of vein was selected, devoid of aneurysms. If this was not possible, previous researchers have suggested needling into the base of an aneurysm. Both needles were always placed retrograde, i.e. away from the fingers. Patients with existing and newly formed fistulas were included in the study. Patients with a newly formed fistula, deemed ready for needling and randomized to BH, started using the BioHole peg immediately to develop BHs. These were placed by the dedicated track former after approximately 5 min of the access achieving hemostasis at the end of dialysis, following removal of the sharp fistula needles see fig. 3 which clearly shows the impression left by the pegs after one week of use. BioHole pegs were used a minimum of 6 times (2 weeks) during the clinical trial; however, experience now suggests that once the sites start to appear 'rounded', cannulation with blunt needles is likely to be successful (which may be within 1–2 weeks or longer).

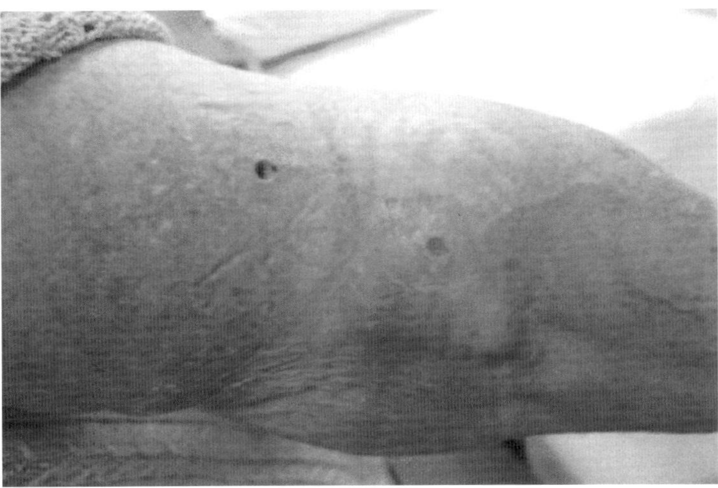

**Fig. 3.** Buttonholes – first week.

Once patients in the BH group had made the transition to blunt needles, they were dialyzed using 15-gauge blunt needles and other competent staff members continued the needling practice. Results from this randomized controlled trial suggested benefit for patients using the BH method for fistula survival, fewer vascular access interventions were needed (fistuloplasty for stenosis or successful thrombectomy), and less enlargement of an existing aneurysm [13].

## Practice Guidelines

The main guidelines for developing BHs in a new patient include identifying the skilled track former (primary cannulator) who can commit to the cannulation for the subsequent 3 weeks (or in combination with a buddy); infection control by following strict hygiene/disinfection practices during hand washing, preparation of equipment, cannulation process, peg insertion, etc., and teaching the patient good hygiene behavior; aseptic insertion and removal of the BioHole peg and teaching the patient to care for the access site while the peg is in situ (keep pegs clean, covered, and dry/avoid tasks which might cause peg dislodgement); close monitoring of early BH development by way of maintaining records/diagrams/photographs, and asking for assistance/advice if experiencing difficulties.

Staff that experience difficulties with cannulation are advised to record the issues and ask for help from an experienced dialysis colleague. Access surveillance is key to a successful program – access function is recorded electronically on 'daily access checks' where there are drop-down lists to insert information about ease of

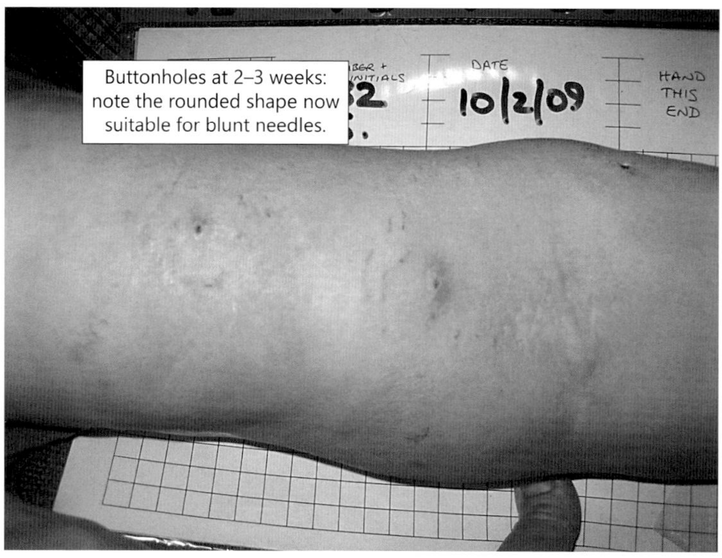


**Fig. 4.** BHs at 2–3 weeks.

needling, needling method used, infection risk (using validated Visual Infusion Phlebitis scoring), and other complications. All patients with a new fistula have their fistula mapped on a chart showing vessels/direction of flow, depth, advice on needle gauge, and required level of competency of the cannulator. The fistula is graded as easy/moderate/difficult and a staff member is accordingly assigned to develop that access. A dedicated access nurse can be consulted whenever difficult cannulation situations arise. Tools to assist include a hand-held ultrasound SonoSite to scan the AVF and measure its diameter and depth. Most large renal centers are now able to access radiology services for ongoing AVF support.

Staff should make a mapping plan for every patient who has a new fistula. This should include instructions about needle size, blood flow rates, maximum flow rate, notes and grade of the cannulator, depth, angle, direction, and packing required with the cannulation method. Staff may need to be encouraged to do this. Staff can sometimes forget to make a careful assessment before attempting cannulation although it is a vital step for successful cannulation. Coordination with the access nurse before the first cannulation may be helpful.

After gaining experience from research subjects, the staff can now attempt to make the transition to blunt needles after three times (1 week) of using the peg. If the blunt needle is not successfully inserted, a sharp needle is again used, the site re-pegged after dialysis, and a blunt needle is attempted at the following dialysis session. Most patients are established on blunt needles within 2 weeks which typically shows buttonholes that appear rounded and are likely to accept blunt needles (see fig. 4). A group discussion by researchers from around the world [7] concluded that the prolonged use of sharp needles in the BH track is thought to lead to complications such as infiltration and excessive bleeding if the track is cut or stretched by the sharp needle, cause damage to the intima of the vessel wall, and may subsequently lead to stenosis and aneurysm formation. The development of spare BH sites is thought to be useful in case difficulties in cannulation are encountered and can give the original sites a rest. Data about peg use and BH progress are recorded on an access sheet until cannulation is well established. In 2014 the majority of patients receiving dialysis at this hospital now successfully use the BH method of cannulation with the BioHole peg to aid in the development of sites. A home HD training program has been offered since 2012, which fits well with the BH program as willing patients are taught to self-cannulate.

## Discussion

In 2005, when cannulation techniques and fistula use were being addressed locally, there was no accepted best practice for the cannulation of AVFs. Our own patients were invited to give their views about current needling practice via service evaluation and it was enlightening to learn that their main concerns were often the unsightly appearance of the fistula ('looks like slugs on my arm') and the time delay in leaving their dialysis chair, after HD, if the fistula took more than a few minutes to achieve hemostasis. It seems that patients just want to get on to dialysis and then off and home as soon as they can, which is understandable. Interestingly, pain was much further down their list of complaints. In view of the increasingly reported observational evidence in favor of the BH technique and with a supportive renal team, this change in practice has taken a big step.

It is interesting to consider and analyze potential barriers that may hinder innovation or limit the implementation of change. HD units often operate using a culture of traditional working practice ('the dialysis factory') where the aim seems to be to get the patients on and off dialysis as quickly as possible due to the pressures of the next shift of patients waiting for treatment. One should really consider if this represents best practice. In the rush of getting the work done, perhaps we should pause for a few moments and ask ourselves if we ever reflect on the way we practice? Cannulation is a task almost always delegated to renal nurses by the medical staff. One may ask how often we critically question what we do. Nurses can be steeped in practice that is based on ritualistic traditional practice even though reflective patient-centered care is often the adopted model.

A main advantage of using the BioHole device is that it allows the track to be created quickly as scar tissue is built. One may question if this is really necessary. Some may disagree, but if you create a tunnel with sharp needles only, it may take longer [5, 6] or cause more problems such as infiltration and hematomas leading to vessel stenosis and aneurysm formation [7]. Presentations have suggested six punctures with sharp needles is enough time to create the track. In reality this is more likely to be 12–15 times. There is nothing wrong with this, it only takes time. If the team of nurses is very big, this can also influence the time factor which may be even longer. However, it is always recommended that the same person perform the cannulation until the track is fully formed [4].

Although using the BioHole peg to help form the BH tracks may be perceived as expensive by adding cost, they may help speed up the transition to blunt needles, which needs to be considered in cost/benefit analysis. Health care workers consider using blunt-ended fistula needles to be safer due to the reduced risk of incurring a needle stick injury during handling of the needle [15].

Patient views about using the pegs and BH method are generally favorable due to improved body image and shorter bleeding times, and patients like to exercise choice by learning to undertake their own needling and be in charge of a task that previously may have left them feeling anxious and disempowered [15]. Staff experience is similar with most expressing a preference for BH [15]. Renal staff turnover can be rapid and there are reports that newer staff can feel apprehensive about using sharp needles for cannulation after experiencing cannulation with blunt needles/BH method.

However, improvements in vascular access survival should not be at the cost to the patient of increased mortality risk by acquiring a life-threatening infection. Disinfection guidelines and infection control measures should be closely followed during any method of vascular access puncture. Due to the reported increased sepsis rates related to BH seen by some centers [7, 15–17], this should warn all practitioners to be ever vigilant in hygiene measures especially around scab removal, needle insertion/removal, and peg insertion. In order to minimize the risk of infection, practice guidelines during BH cannulation should follow enhanced care as used when accessing a fistula graft or central venous catheter line. Ongoing monitoring and audit for vascular access infection is recommended [16]. It is well reported (social media, patient blogs, and YouTube footage) that patients who are self-caring often resort to shortcuts in their technique. This should be addressed by the home therapies team. The nursing staff should also attend regular mandatory infection control updates and refresher training to maintain good BH technique.

Success with the BioHole peg device has been recognized by another team who are currently researching the development of an alternative needling aid. The SAVE study has reported benefits including a 100% AVF survival rate at 6 months in 51 patients using a titanium device that is surgically implanted beneath the skin and directly attached to the fistula wall [18]. This acts as a subcutaneous needle guide and has been aimed to help practitioners use the BH method to cannulate more difficult fistulas (e.g. in obese patients). Addressing comorbidities that give rise to associated vascular access problems in patients requiring HD is a constant challenge. Manufacturers of the BioHole peg device are addressing the challenge of patients with deep vessels or superfluous tissue and are now making pegs available in longer lengths than the standard 5 mm.

## Conclusions

The BH cannulation method using the BioHole peg device offers considerable advantages including reduced risk of cannulation complications and AVF failure, speedy transition to blunt needles, the tunnel track remaining narrow thus reducing risk of developing an exit site infection, and suitability in patients with comorbidities and difficult sites. Possible associated disadvantages may include the increased cost for purchasing BioHole pegs during the track break-in period and potential complications associated with use of the peg such as discomfort, bleeding, and risk of infection. These risks/disadvantages minimize after the transition to blunt needles which in itself is a safer option than using sharp needles. As supported by KDOQI and the UK Renal Association, adoption of BH as the cannulation technique of choice is recommended in the majority of HD patients with a native fistula.

## Relevance to Practice

Implementing a successful new cannulation method will only be achieved through a lot of hard work and dedication from the whole health care professional team as well as the patients. Patient experience has been enhanced as patients using BH now benefit from an access that is generally not unsightly and often hardly noticeable, that causes little or no pain or anxiety during the cannulation process, and that quickly stops bleeding once the needles are removed. Patients will have to 'work with the staff' during this time of change and learn to be a 'patient' patient. Patients are empowered to learn to self-cannulate and can even work towards managing their own HD at home. For staff, using innovation to improve care develops their skills, critical thinking, and job satisfaction. Renal health care professionals should be encouraged to look at other areas of practice where patient experience/survival can be improved. The author warmly acknowledges the collaboration with renal colleagues and the patients at the Royal Berkshire Hospital during this study in cannulation practice and for the on-going research and development across the renal community.

## References

1 National Kidney Foundation KDOQI: Vascular Access Guidelines 2006. http:www.kidney. org/professionals/KDOQI/guideline_upHD_ PD_VA/hd_guide1.html.
2 British Renal Society, UK Renal Association: The Fifth Edition of the Clinical Practice Guidelines. Vascular Access for Haemodialysis. Final Version (January 5, 2011). http:// www.renal.org/home.
3 Twardowski Z, Kubara H: Different sites versus constant sites of needle insertion into arteriovenous fistulas for treatment by repeated dialysis. Dial Transplant 1979;8:978–980.
4 Ball L: Improving arteriovenous fistula cannulation skills. Nephrol Nurs J 2005;32:611–617.
5 Struthers J, Allan A, Peel RK, et al: Buttonhole needling of arteriovenous fistulae: a randomised controlled trial. ASAIO J 2010;56: 319–322.
6 Milburn J, Macaulay E, Annand J, et al: Fistula cannulation – the buttonhole method. Br J Ren Med 2008;13:4–7.
7 Murcutt G: Buttonhole cannulation: should this become the default technique for dialysis patients with native fistulas? Summary of the EDTNA/ERCA Journal Club discussion Autumn 2007. J Ren Care 2008;34:101–108.
8 Toma S, Shinzato T, Fukui H, et al: A time-saving method to create a fixed puncture route for the buttonhole technique. Nephrol Dial Transplant 2003;18:2118–2121.
9 King J: Implementing the buttonhole method using the BioHole peg in a busy dialysis unit: a report of the development of current practice. J Ren Care 2009;35:192–200.
10 Marticorena RM, Hunter J, Macleod S, et al: Use of the BioHole™ device for the creation of tunnel tracks for buttonhole cannulation of fistula for hemodialysis. Hemodial Int 2011;15:243–249.
11 Marticorena RM, Hunter J, Macleod S, et al: The salvage of aneurysmal fistulae utilizing a modified buttonhole cannulation technique and multiple cannulators. Hemodial Int 2006; 10:193–200.
12 Sucker A, Schatzle-Schuler G, Pankiewicz T, et al: Constant site needle insertion versus different site needle insertion into the Cimino Brescia fistula. Proc EDTNA 1984;13:59–66.
13 Vaux E, King J, Lloyd S, et al: Effect of buttonhole cannulation with a polycarbonate peg on in-center hemodialysis outcomes: a randomized controlled trial. Am J Kidney Dis 2013;62:81–88.
14 Parisotto M, Schoder V, Miriunis C, et al: Cannulation technique influences arteriovenous fistula and graft survival. Kidney Int 2014;86:790–797.
15 Ball L, Treat L, Riffle V, et al: A multi-center perspective of the buttonhole technique in the Pacific Northwest. Nephrol Nurs J 2007; 34:234–241.
16 MacRae JM, Ahmed SB, Atkar R, et al: A randomized trial comparing buttonhole with rope ladder needling in conventional hemodialysis patients. Clin J Am Soc Nephrol 2012;7:1632–1638.
17 Atkar RK, MacRae JM: The buttonhole technique for fistula cannulation: pros and cons. Curr Opin Nephrol Hypertens 2013;22:629–636.
18 Jennings W, Galt S, Shenoy S, et al: The Venous Window Needle Guide, a hemodialysis cannulation device for salvage of uncannulatable arteriovenous fistulas. J Vasc Surg 2014; 60:1024–1032.

Jennie King, RN, BSc (Hons)
42 Shaw Way, Mountbatten
Plymouth PL9 9XH (UK)
E-Mail jennieking2013@gmail.com

Misra M, Toma S, Shinzato T (eds): Buttonhole Cannulation: Current Prospects and Challenges.
Contrib Nephrol. Basel, Karger, 2015, vol 186, pp 33–40 (DOI: 10.1159/000431161)

# Causes and Solutions of the Trampoline Effect

Masamiki Miwa[a] · Noboru Ota[a] · Chiyono Ando[b] ·
Yukio Miyazaki[c]

[a]Atsuta Clinic, Nagoya, and [b]Michishirube, and [c]Miyazaki Ladies Clinic, Gifu, Japan

## Abstract

A trampoline effect may occur mainly when a buttonhole tract and the vessel flap fail to
form a straight line. Certain findings, however, suggest another cause is when the vessel
flap is too small. The frequency of the trampoline effect, for example, is lower when a buttonhole tract is created by multiple punctures of the arteriovenous fistula (AVF) vessel
than when it is done by one-time puncture of the vessel. Lower frequency of the trampoline effect with multiple punctures of the AVF vessel may be due to enlargement of the
initial puncture hole on the vessel every time the vessel is punctured with a sharp needle.
Even if aiming at exactly the same point on the AVF vessel every time, the actual puncture
point shifts slightly at every puncture, which potentially results in enlargement of the initial hole on the AVF vessel. Moreover, in some patients, continued use of a buttonhole
tract for an extended period of time increases the frequency of the trampoline effect. In
such cases, reduction of the incidence of the trampoline effect can be achieved by one
buttonhole cannulation using a new dull needle with sharp side edges that is used to enlarge the vessel flap. Such single buttonhole cannulation may suggest that the increased
frequency of the trampoline effect also potentially occurs in association with gradually
diminishing flap size. As a final observation, dull needle insertion into a vessel flap in the
reverse direction has been more smoothly achieved than insertion into a vessel flap in the
conventional direction. A vessel flap in the reverse direction can be adopted clinically.

© 2015 S. Karger AG, Basel

One of the most important issues with the buttonhole method may be the in-
ability of a dull needle to reach the arteriovenous fistula (AVF) vessel wall
through a buttonhole tract to drop into the vessel lumen (i.e. trampoline effect).
The trampoline effect may occur mainly when a buttonhole tract and a vessel

flap fail to form a straight line due to a shift of the flap caused by an involuntary, slight twist of the forearm. Recent findings, however, suggest another cause of the phenomenon is when a vessel flap is too small. Therefore, in this article we discuss the relationship between vessel flap size and the trampoline effect, and then suggest solutions for the trampoline effect.

## Trampoline Effect Frequency and the Buttonhole Tract Creation Method

*The Frequency of the Trampoline Effect in Japan and Other Countries*
The buttonhole method has not been adopted widely in Japan. Marked high frequency of the trampoline effect mainly explains the low prevalence of the buttonhole method in Japan. Nakahara [1], for example, reported that the trampoline effect occurred at a rate of 50.9% at her hospital. However, the frequency at Nakahara's hospital appeared comparatively low among hospitals in Japan. The trampoline effect occurs at a rate of 90% or higher at many Japanese hospitals according to our private communications. In contrast, the frequency of the trampoline effect is much lower in other countries. According to the 'Summary of the EDTNA/ERCA Journal Club discussion Autumn 2007', Jackie Ross and Jacqui Annand reported that approximately 24% of patients experience the trampoline effect [2].

*The Reason for the High Frequency of the Trampoline Effect in Japan*
The method of buttonhole tract creation at many facilities in Japan varies from the method used in other countries. In Japan, cannulation using a sharp needle to create a buttonhole tract is performed in the first hemodialysis session only [3]. In subsequent hemodialysis sessions, buttonhole cannulation is performed using a dull needle. This method involves creating a single arc-shaped incision (i.e. flap) in the AVF vessel, whose chord is smaller than the diameter of the sharp needle used to create the flap. When a silicone sheet was punctured obliquely with a 17-gauge sharp needle at a 30° angle, the length (1.27 mm) of the chord of the arc-shaped incision was 86% of the outer diameter (1.47 mm) of the sharp needle used to create the incision. One can easily imagine the difficulty in inserting a dull-needle into such a small flap formed from one puncture in the AVF vessel wall by using a sharp needle.

In other countries, on the other hand, cannulation using sharp needles is performed 8–12 times to create a buttonhole tract, and upon creating a buttonhole tract, a dull needle is subsequently inserted [4, 5]. However, when puncturing the AVF vessel 8–12 times using a sharp needle, even experienced hemodialysis staff may not be able puncture exactly the same point of the vessel in every session. At each puncture, the puncture point may shift slightly so that the size of the puncture hole gradually increases. If so, a larger puncture hole may form in the vascular wall when puncturing multiple times with a sharp needle than when puncturing only one time to create a buttonhole tract. As a result, when puncturing the vessel multiple times with a sharp needle to create a buttonhole tract, a lower incidence of the trampoline effect may result.

*Comparison of Trampoline Effect Frequency between Multiple Punctures and a Single Puncture to Create a Buttonhole Tract*
To confirm the hypothesis mentioned above, we compared consequences in terms of the trampoline effect occurrence between 9 patients in whom a buttonhole tract was newly established by puncturing the AVF vessel with sharp needles during six consecutive hemodialysis sessions and 24 patients in whom such a tract had been created previously by puncturing the vessel with a sharp needle at only one hemodialysis session.

In the patients whose AVF vessels were punctured with sharp needles during six consecutive hemodialysis sessions, the trampoline effect occurred at a rate of 22% for 3 months following the establishment of the buttonhole tract. In contrast, for 19 of the 24 patients (79%) who had been punctured previously with a sharp needle at only one hemodialysis session, buttonhole cannulation had been abandoned within 2 weeks from the creation of the buttonhole tract because of a trampoline effect occurring too frequently. Due to the patients' wishes, buttonhole cannulation was discontinued for the remaining 5 patients (21%) within 1 month of the creation of the buttonhole tract. In these patients, more time had been required for dull needle cannulation because of the trampoline effect.

## Increased Frequency of the Trampoline Effect Due to a Diminished Vessel Flap

*Vessel Flap Diminishing Over Time*
When a buttonhole tract is used for an extended period of time, the frequency of the trampoline effect increases in some patients. Currently, the reason for this phenomenon is not clear, but it may occur because the vascular flap narrows over time.

*Restoration Needle*
A special dull needle (Kamada Spring Co., Ltd., Saitama, Japan) was developed for widening the vessel flap that narrows over a long periods of use [6]. Until an official name is decided on, we will refer to this puncture needle as a restoration needle.

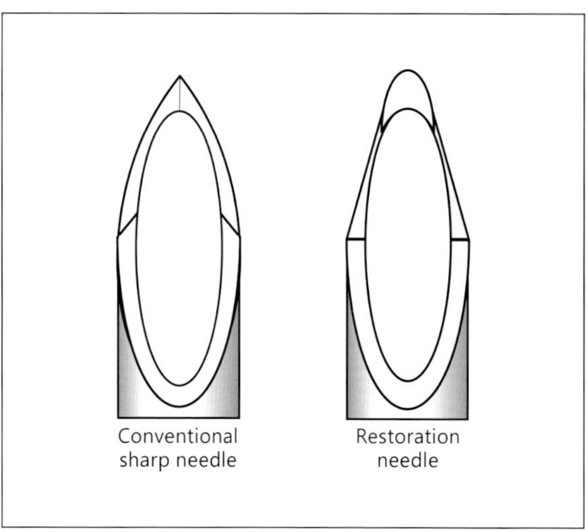


**Fig. 1.** Schematic diagrams of a conventional sharp needle (left diagram) and restoration needle (right diagram). With a conventional sharp needle, both side edges are sharp blades, and the tip is a sharp point. With the restoration needle, both side edges are sharp blades, but the tip is dull.

In figure 1, the left side shows a schematic diagram of a conventional sharp needle, and the right side shows a schematic diagram of a restoration needle. As seen in the left diagram, both side edges of the conventional sharp needle have sharp blades from the tip to the front that are approximately one third of the bevel. As a result, the tip of a conventional sharp needle is a sharp point.

In contrast, as shown on the right in figure 1, the restoration needle has a dull tip and only the edges, not including the tip portion, are sharp blades up to approximately one third of the bevel. When this restoration needle is inserted into the vessel flap that has narrowed through a buttonhole tract, the blade parts of the edge cut and widen the narrowed flap.

*Clinical Effectiveness of Vessel Flap Enlargement Using a Restoration Needle*
As of April 1, 2013, among 83 patients, nurses reported 9 patients in whom the trampoline effect occurred more frequently than in the past. These 9 patients had been on hemodialysis for 58.5 ± 21.9 months on average, and the average length since the creation of the buttonhole tract was 37.2 ± 8.6 months. In all cases, a 17-gauge dull needle was used for buttonhole cannulation.

For these 9 patients, buttonhole cannulation was performed using a restoration needle at a certain hemodialysis session to widen the potentially diminishing vessel flap. As a result, the frequency of the trampoline effect decreased from 38.2% for 3 months before widening of the vessel flap with the restoration needle to 19.5% for 3 months after cannulation with the restoration needle.



Miwa · Ota · Ando · Miyazaki

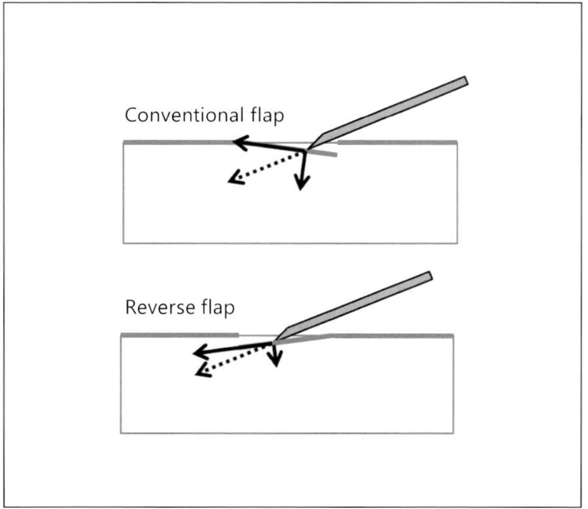



**Fig. 2.** Pressing forces acting upon the flaps in the conventional (upper diagram) and reverse directions (lower diagram). With the flap in the conventional direction, due to the component of the force pushing the flap toward its base, the tip of the dull needle easily passes over the flap.

## Directions of the Arteriovenous Fistula Vessel Flap and Smoother Entry of a Dull Needle into the Vessel Lumen

*Vessel Flap in the Conventional Direction*

If a vessel flap is in the conventional direction, and the insertion angle of a dull needle is too narrow, the tip of the needle may easily go over the vessel flap. On the other hand, if the insertion angle is too wide, the tip of the needle might cut the vessel flap.

When the tip of the dull needle pushes a flap in the conventional direction obliquely, as shown on the left in figure 2, the pressing force acting upon the flap can be resolved into a component pushing the flap toward its base and a component turning the flap down into the AVF vessel lumen. Due to the component of the force pushing the flap toward its base, the tip of the dull needle easily passes over the flap before the needle can turn the flap down into the vessel lumen.

To prevent this from occurring, when the tip of the dull needle reaches the vessel flap, we involuntarily enlarge the insertion angle on the vessel until the dull needle drops into the vessel lumen through the vessel flap.

*Vessel Flap in the Reverse Direction*

This problem of the insertion angle of a dull needle could be readily solved by creation of a reverse-directional vessel flap. As shown on the right in figure 2, when the tip of the dull needle pushes a reverse-directional flap obliquely, the pressing force acting upon the flap can be resolved into a component pushing the flap toward its tip and a component turning the flap down into the vessel

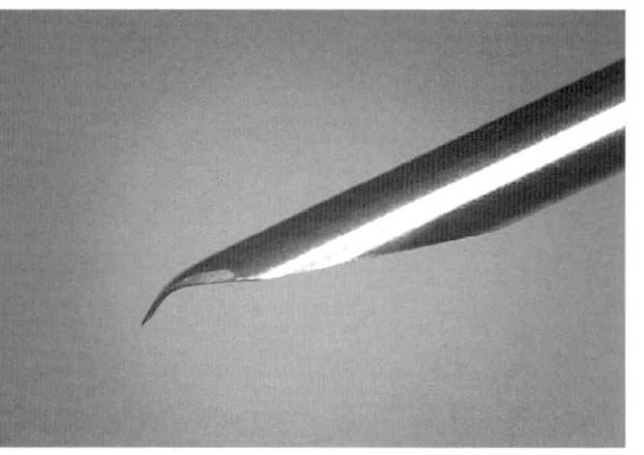

**Fig. 3.** Schematic diagrams of a new needle to form a vessel flap in the reverse direction. The needle is used to puncture an AVF vessel at approximately 30°, with the bevel facing downwards.

lumen. Therefore, with a reverse-directional flap, the tip of the dull needle drops into the AVF vessel as if dropping down a slide. Thus, the vessel flap in the reverse direction facilitates smoother entry of a dull needle into the vessel lumen in buttonhole cannulation.

### Needles Forming a Flap in the Reverse Direction

In order to create a buttonhole tract and a vessel flap with the tip forward and the base backward with respect to the dull needle insertion direction, we used a new sharp needle (Kamada Spring Co., Ltd., Saitama, Japan). The needle is characterized by the bevel point curved toward the needle lumen, as shown in figure 3. The length of the curved segment was 0.66 mm, and the curvature radius was 1.63 mm. The outer diameter of this needle is 1.47 mm (17 G). In the following, we refer to this as a curved-point needle.

The curved-point needle is used to puncture an AVF vessel at about a 30° angle, with the bevel facing downwards. When the needle tip reaches the vessel wall with its bevel downwards, the curved segment of the bevel penetrates the vessel wall at the same angle.

### Displacement of Flap with Insertion of a Dull Needle

To better understand the reason for smoother insertion of a dull needle into the flap in the reverse direction, we created flaps in the conventional and reverse directions on a silicone sheet and compared displacement of each flap when a dull needle was inserted.

When a dull needle was inserted into the conventional directional flap, as shown on the left in figure 4, the flap was folded back nearly 150° on the back of the sheet and was situated on the upper surface of the cylindrical portion of the dull needle. With the reverse directional flap, however, the flap only bent about 30° on the back of the sheet and stuck along the lower surface of the cylindrical portion of the dull needle, as shown on the right in figure 4. These results indicate that with a vessel flap in the reverse direction, the tip of the dull needle enters the AVF vessel as if moving down a slide.

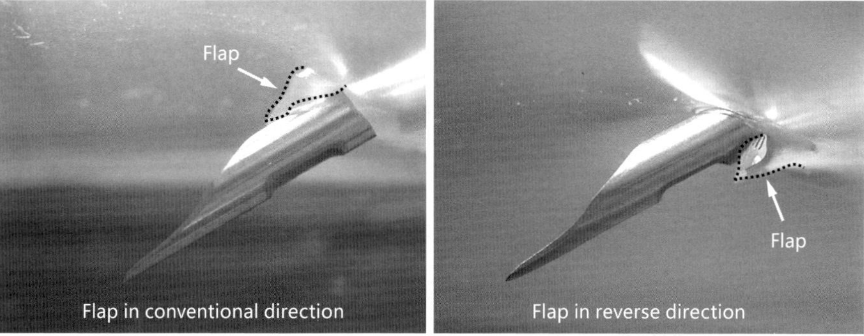


**Fig. 4.** Displacement of a flap when a dull needle is inserted. With the flap in the conventional direction, the flap was folded back nearly 150° on the back of the silicone (left diagram). With the flap in the reverse direction, the flap only bent approximately 30° on the back of the sheet (right diagram).

### *Clinical Comparison of Conventional and Reverse Direction Flaps for Ease of Buttonhole Cannulation*

In order to evaluate the vessel flaps clinically in terms of buttonhole cannulation difficulty, we selected 16 patients who had an AVF with native vessels. All of the patients wanted AVF vessel cannulation by the buttonhole technique. These patients were randomly assigned to a group with the vessel flaps in the conventional direction or to a group with the vessel flaps in the reverse direction.

As a result, among the 8 patients with the vessel flaps in the conventional direction, 4 patients reported some sort of discomfort when inserting a dull needle into the vessel lumen. In contrast, among the 8 patients with the vessel flaps in the reverse direction, none claimed such discomfort when inserting a dull needle into the vessel lumen. Moreover, all staff responsible for buttonhole cannulation stated that needle insertion into the flap in the reverse direction was more smoothly achieved than into the flap in the conventional direction.

## Conclusions

Puncture of the same point of the AVF vessel with sharp needles at multiple hemodialysis sessions is important not only for establishment of a buttonhole tract, but also for creation of a larger vessel flap that prevents the trampoline effect. When a buttonhole tract continues to be used for an extended period of time, frequency of the trampoline effect increases in some patients. Such increased frequency can be corrected by performing one buttonhole cannulation with a new, dull-tip needle with sharp side edges. Dull needle insertion into the flap in the reverse direction is more smoothly achieved than insertion into the flap in the conventional direction.

## References

1 Nakahara N: Difficulty in buttonhole needling and its solving method (abstract). J Jpn Soc Dial Ther 2007;40(suppl):339.
2 Murcutt G: Buttonhole cannulation: should this become the default technique for dialysis patients with native fistulas? Summary of the EDTNA/ERCA Journal Club discussion Autumn 2007. J Ren Care 2008;34:101–108.
3 Ogawa C, Okada K, Iijima S, et al: The buttonhole method using single needling. J Jpn Soc Dial Ther 2010;43:989–992.
4 Twardowski Z: Different sites versus constant sites of needle insertion into arteriovenous fistulas for treatment by repeated dialysis. Dial Transpl 1979;8:978–980.
5 Twardowski ZJ: Buttonhole method for needle insertion into A-V fistula. Nephrol Dial Pol 2006;10:156–158.
6 Toma S: New method to prevent trampoline effect (abstract). 7th Congr Int Soc Hemodial, Ginowan City, 2014, p 60.


Masamiki Miwa, MD
Atsuta Clinic
61-3 Hibino-cho, Atsuta-ku, Nagoya-shi
Aichi 456-0074 (Japan)
E-Mail miwamasamiki@gmail.com

Misra M, Toma S, Shinzato T (eds): Buttonhole Cannulation: Current Prospects and Challenges.
Contrib Nephrol. Basel, Karger, 2015, vol 186, pp 41–47 (DOI: 10.1159/000431166)

# A New Method That Enables Complete Removal of Scabs at Buttonhole Entry Sites

Takahiro Shinzato[a] · Masatomi Sasaki[a] · Noboru Ota[b] ·
Kazuhiko Shibata[c] · Hiroyoshi Fukui[d] · Shigeki Toma[e] ·
Kenji Maeda[a]

[a] Daiko Medical Engineering Research Institute, and [b] Atsuta Clinic, Nagoya, [c] Yokohama-Minami
Clinic, Yokohama, [d] Chuo-Jin Clinic, Kumamoto, and [e] Toma Clinic, Nishihara-cho, Japan

## Abstract

***Background:*** Scab removal is a time-consuming process and often injures the skin at a
buttonhole entry site. Incomplete removal of scabs may cause access-related infection.
***Methods:*** In a new procedure, buttonhole entry sites were treated with a moist healing
step after hemodialysis, and then a formed scab was wiped off with a microfiber towel
during bathing on the night prior to hemodialysis, which was performed on the following
day. In the moist healing step, the entry site was disinfected with a diluted povidone-iodine solution (0.1% povidone-iodine solution). ***Results:*** When the buttonhole entry sites
of the patients were treated with the new procedure, the scabs had already been removed
at the buttonhole entry sites, and the sites were covered with a thin transparent membrane. Histological examination showed the thin membrane was stratum corneum, in
which nuclei are still seen in keratinocytes. ***Conclusion:*** By treating the buttonhole entry
sites of patients with the wound moist healing method and then rubbing the sites with a
microfiber towel during bathing, scabs can be removed without injuring the skin at the
sites in advance. © 2015 S. Karger AG, Basel

Scab removal is a time-consuming process performed immediately before buttonhole cannulation. Scab removal using a sharp needle often injures the skin at
a buttonhole entry site and causes pain to patients. Moreover, even if complete
removal of a scab is attempted, small fractions of a scab potentially remain at the
buttonhole entry site. Such small scab fractions may cause access-related infection [1–3].

As a solution to these concerns relating to the current scab removal method, we have devised a new treatment procedure. The procedure involves treatment of a buttonhole entry site after hemodialysis with a moist healing step and then wiping off formed scabs with a microfiber towel during bathing on the night prior to hemodialysis, which was performed on the following day. In this chapter, details of this new entry site treatment procedure are described, together with its clinical outcomes.

## Methods

*Patients*
The new entry site treatment procedure was applied to 26 patients (10 males and 16 females, mean age ± SD: 66 ± 4 years). The etiology of kidney disease in various patients was chronic nephritis in 3, diabetic nephropathy in 7, nephrosclerosis in 3, and uncertain in 13 patients. All patients were on maintenance hemodialysis therapy using a native arteriovenous fistula and were dialyzed 3 times a week. Their buttonhole tracts were 7.3 ± 4.7 months old, and the patients had been on hemodialysis for 24.8 ± 9.7 months at the time the new procedure was introduced.

*New Entry Site Treatment Procedure*
Disinfectant
A 0.1% povidone-iodine solution (diluted povidone-iodine solution) was used to disinfect the buttonhole entry site before, during, and after hemodialysis. The 0.1% povidone-iodine solution was prepared by diluting commercially available 10% povidone-iodine solution 100-fold with sterile distilled water.

Disinfection of the Buttonhole Entry Sites before and during Hemodialysis
Before buttonhole cannulation, no scabs were to be present at the entry sites (described later). The entry sites were promptly disinfected with 0.1% povidone-iodine solution. After dull needles were cannulated and fixed on the skin surface, the entry sites were covered with cotton pads soaked in 0.1% povidone-iodine solution during hemodialysis.

Disinfection of the Buttonhole Entry Site after Hemodialysis
After the dull needles were removed and any bleeding was stopped, the entry sites were disinfected with the 0.1% povidone-iodine solution.

Moist Healing Step
Film dressings of 16 × 29 mm (Careleaves®; Nichiban Co., Ltd., Tokyo, Japan) were applied to the buttonhole entry sites immediately after disinfecting the entry sites after hemodialysis. Patients were instructed to remove the film dressings 24 h after the dressings were applied.

Scab Removal
Patients were instructed to wipe off the created scabs using a microfiber towel while bathing the night before the next hemodialysis.

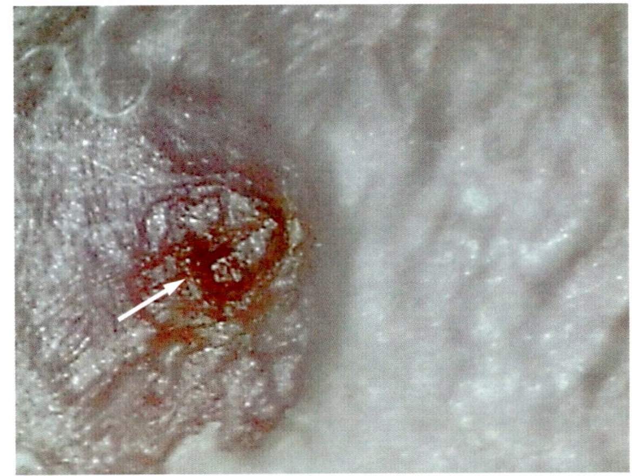

**Fig. 1.** Enlarged photograph of the buttonhole entry site of the patient treated with the new procedure. The photograph, magnified ×25, was taken before the next hemodialysis. The opening of the buttonhole tract appeared red through the membrane (indicated by the arrow).

*Clinical Outcomes*

Two of the patients were asked to visit their respective facility prior to taking a bath in order to examine whether scabs were created at the buttonhole entry sites. The request to visit the respective facilities was between 2 and 3 weeks after the start of the new entry site treatment procedure.

In addition, when each patient visited their facility for hemodialysis, a photograph of the entry site, magnified 25 times, was taken with a microscope digital camera (3RVIETER500UV®; 3R Systems Co., Ltd., Fukuoka, Japan) between 2 and 3 weeks after the start of the new entry site treatment procedure. On these enlarged photographs, appearance of the buttonhole entry sites was observed.

In 2 patients who gave informed consent, the thin membrane that formed at the buttonhole entry site of each patient was peeled off with tweezers for histological examination when the patients visited the facility for hemodialysis. The specimens were stained with hematoxylin-eosin pigment and placed onto a slide, which was prepared for observation under a microscope.

## Results

*Scab Formation Prior to Bathing*

When the 2 patients visited the facility, smaller scabs were observed at the entry site of each patient before the patients bathed. The scabs were elliptical and round.

*Observation of the Entry Sites before the Next Hemodialysis*

According to the enlarged photographs, no scab was found at the entry site of either patient before the next hemodialysis. The sites were covered with a thin transparent membrane, and the opening of the buttonhole tracts appeared red through the membrane (portion indicated by the arrow in fig. 1).

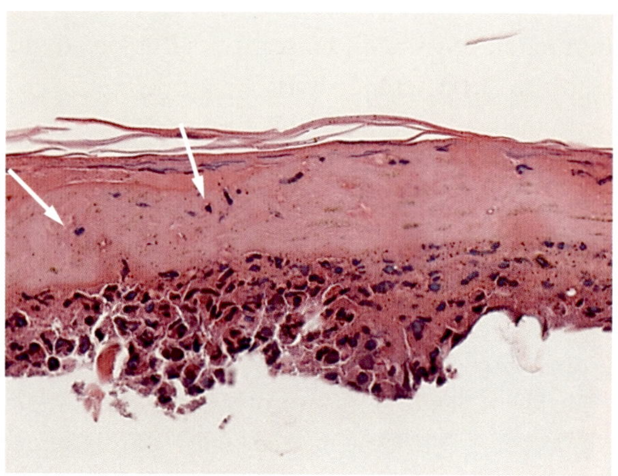

**Fig. 2.** Microscopic appearance of thin membrane formed at the buttonhole entry sites (hematoxylin-eosin stain, ×200). Histological examination showed the thin membrane was stratum corneum, in which nuclei are still seen in keratinocytes (indicated by the arrows).

*Histological Examination of the Membrane*

Histological examination showed that the thin membrane formed at the buttonhole entry site was stratum corneum (fig. 2). In the stratum corneum, nuclei were still seen in keratinocytes, indicating that enucleation of keratinocytes was incomplete (i.e. parakeratosis).

Beneath the stratum corneum, fibrin deposits were observed. In the fibrin deposits, neutrophils were observed that are thought to have been included in the original leaked components.

## Discussion

Our new treatment procedure of the buttonhole entry sites will shorten the time required for buttonhole cannulation because scabs are removed in advance on the night prior to hemodialysis, which is performed the following day. In the scab removal step of the new procedure, the removal of scabs does not injure the skin at the buttonhole entry sites or cause pain to patients. The reason for the lack of injury or discomfort is because the scabs are wiped off with a microfiber towel and not picked off with a sharp needle. The reason for easier scab removal in this method is because the scabs are smaller in size due to the moist healing approach and softened by absorbing water during bathing. Recently, Hadley and Moran [4] also showed that softening scabs by water absorption makes scab removal easier. They used gauze soaked with warm tap water over each scab for 20 min to soften the scab.

When the buttonhole entry sites were treated with this new procedure, the sites were almost completely healed before the next hemodialysis. At the buttonhole entry sites, no scabs were observed, but stratum corneum formed before the next hemodialysis.

In the keratinocytes of this stratum corneum, nuclei were still observed (i.e. parakeratosis). Parakeratosis indicates that turnover of the stratum corneum is accelerated [5]. General cornification is not completed in 2–3 days, but in parakeratosis, cornification can be completed in a shorter time (e.g. 1 day). Based on these facts, this stratum corneum is likely to have formed within 1 day beneath the scab. This rapid formation of the stratum corneum in our patients may be due to the moist healing approach.

In the moist healing step of the new entry site treatment procedure, a buttonhole entry site is disinfected before, during, and after hemodialysis. Disinfection, however, is avoided with the conventional wound moist healing method because it hinders healing of a wound. Nevertheless, avoidance of disinfection is thought to be dangerous in the case of the buttonhole cannulation technique. A buttonhole tract is at potential risk of infection from bacterial growth because the space represents a type of fistula filled with protein-containing fluid between the skin surface and the vessel wall.

As a disinfectant, 0.1% povidone-iodine solution (i.e. diluted povidone-iodine solution) was used in our modified moist healing step. It is reported that 0.1% povidone-iodine solution has a greater bactericidal activity than 10% povidone-iodine solution (i.e. undiluted povidone-iodine solution) [6] because the concentration of free molecular iodine is paradoxically 10 times higher in 0.1% povidone-iodine solution than in 10% povidone-iodine solution [7]. Free molecular iodine is only an iodine species for which a correlation between concentration and bactericidal activity has been proven [8].

Nevertheless, when the entry sites are disinfected with 0.1% povidone-iodine solution, the concentration of free molecular iodine in the solution applied to the skin surface decreases with time. Such a decrease in concentration is due to consumption by contact with the skin and transfer into the body through the stratum corneum. Due to a shortage of a sustained-release reservoir of available molecular iodine, the concentration of free molecular iodine readily decreases in association with consumption and absorption in diluted povidone-iodine solution. In order to compensate for this disadvantage in the new entry site treatment procedure, after disinfection with 0.1% povidone-iodine solution, the entry sites were covered with cotton pads soaked in 0.1% povidone-iodine solution during hemodialysis.

It has been reported that occlusive dressings help prevent infection by presenting a barrier to potential pathogens [9]. However, covering of entry sites with cotton pads soaked in diluted povidone-iodine solution has not been proven to be a barrier to bacteria. Nevertheless, such cotton pads are likely to prevent bacterial invasion. Free molecular iodine is potentially supplied to the skin surface from the cotton pads soaked in 0.1% povidone-iodine solution while the free molecular iodine is consumed by contact with the skin and absorbed into the body through the stratum corneum.

When comparing the sustained efficacy of disinfection between our method and the conventional method to disinfect sites with undiluted povidone-iodine solution before hemodialysis, our method may be more effective in theory. When the entry sites are covered with cotton pads soaked in diluted povidone-iodine solution, free molecular iodine is potentially supplied continuously to the skin from the cotton pads soaked in diluted povidone-iodine solution. In contrast, when the entry sites are disinfected with undiluted povidone-iodine solution and covered with dry gauzes, povidone-iodine solution soon dries up and loses bacteriocidal activity. In solid povidone-iodine, iodine is present in the form of discrete $HI_3$ [10], which exhibits no bactericidal activity [8].

In the present study, when diluted povidone-iodine solution was used as a disinfectant in the new entry site treatment procedure, stratum corneum successfully formed beneath the scab. Formation may be due to the minimal toxicity of the 0.1% povidone-iodine solution. The cytotoxicity of povidone-iodine solution has been documented in in vitro studies [11–15]. However, the results of in vivo studies suggest that povidone-iodine does not interfere with healing, especially if povidone-iodine is used at concentrations of 0.1% or lower [12–15]. These results contradict the commonly held belief that both toxicity and bactericidal activity of povidone-iodine solution are due to free molecular iodine. The reason for this contraindication is unclear.

In conclusion, we successfully removed scabs without injuring the skin at the buttonhole entry sites on the day prior to hemodialysis. We achieved these results by treating the sites using the wound moist healing method and then rubbing the sites with a microfiber towel during bathing.

## References


1  Gray N: The risk of sepsis from buttonhole needling must be appreciated. Nephrol Dial Transplant 2010;25:2385–2386.
2  Birchenough E, Moore C, Stevens K, et al: Buttonhole cannulation in adult patients on hemodialysis: an increased risk of infection? Nephrol Nurs J 2010;37:491–498.
3  Nesrallah GE, Cuerden M, Wong JH, et al: *Staphylococcus aureus* bacteremia and buttonhole cannulation: long-term safety and efficacy of mupirocin prophylaxis. Clin J Am Soc Nephrol 2010;5:1047–1053.
4  Hadley K, Moran J: Buttonhole access: non-invasive scab removal (abstract): Annual Dialysis Conference, March 2010. Hemodial Int 2010;14:98.
5  Lever WF, Elder DE: Lever's Histopathology of the Skin, ed 9. Philadelphia, Lippincott Williams & Wilkins, 2005.
6  Berkelman RL, Holland BW, Anderson RL: Increased bactericidal activity of dilute preparations of povidone-iodine solutions. J Clin Microbiol 1982;15:635–639.


  Shinzato · Sasaki · Ota · Shibata · Fukui · Toma · Maeda

7 Gottardi W: Potentiometrische Bestimmung der Gleichgewichtskonzentrationen an freiem und komplex gebundenem Iod in wässrigen Lösungen von Polyvinylpyrrolidon-Iod (PVP-Iod) (English abstract). Fresenius Z Anal Chem 1983;314:582–585.

8 Hickey J, Panicucci R, Duan Y, et al: Control of the amount of free molecular iodine in iodine germicides. J Pharm Pharmacol 1997;49: 1195–1199.

9 Hutchinson JJ, Lawrence JC: Wound infection under occlusive dressings. J Hosp Infect 1991;17:83–94.

10 Schenck HU, Simak P, Haedicke E: Structure of polyvinylpyrrolidione-iodine (povidone-iodine). J Pharm Sci 1979;68:1505–1509.

11 Balin AK, Pratt L: Dilute povidone-iodine solutions inhibit human skin fibroblast growth. Dermatol Surg 2002;28:210–214.

12 Naor J, Savion N, Blumenthal M, et al: Corneal endothelial cytotoxicity of diluted povidone-iodine. J Cataract Refract Surg 2001;27: 941–947.

13 Brånemark PI, Albrektsson B, Lindström J, et al: Local tissue effects of wound disinfectants. Acta Chir Scand 1966;357(suppl):166–176.

14 Brennan SS, Leaper DJ: The effect of antiseptics on the healing wound: a study using the rabbit ear chamber. Br J Surg 1985;72:780–782.

15 Brånemark PI, Ekholm R, Albrektsson B, et al: Tissue injury caused by wound disinfectants. J Bone Joint Surg Am 1967;49:48–62.

Takahiro Shinzato, MD, PhD
Daiko Medical Engineering Research Institute
4-16-23 Daiko Higashi-ku Nagoya, Aichi-ken (Japan)
E-Mail shinzato@xj8.so-net.ne.jp

Misra M, Toma S, Shinzato T (eds): Buttonhole Cannulation: Current Prospects and Challenges.
Contrib Nephrol. Basel, Karger, 2015, vol 186, pp 48–56 (DOI: 10.1159/000431164)

# Deformity of Buttonhole Entry Site Causes Higher Frequency of Vascular Access-Related Infection

Shoichi Sato[a] · Takahiro Shinzato[b] · Naoko Sakai[a] ·
Katsuyuki Ohkuri[a] · Masatomi Sasaki[b] · Shigeru Nakai[c] ·
Shigeki Toma[d]

[a]Hino Clinic, Osaka, [b]Daiko Medical Engineering Research Institute, Nagoya, [c]Faculty of Clinical
Engineering, Fujita Health University, Toyoake, and [d]Toma Clinic, Nishihara-cho, Japan

## Abstract

***Background:*** Vascular access-related infection is more frequent in patients using the buttonhole method for cannulation of the arteriovenous access for hemodialysis. Deformity of buttonhole entry sites is frequently observed among patients on the buttonhole method for extended periods of time. With deformed buttonhole entry sites, moreover, scabs are often incompletely removed at the time of buttonhole cannulation. ***Method:*** In 166 patients using the buttonhole method at Hino Clinic in Osaka, Japan as of June 30, 2014, the shapes of buttonhole entry sites were categorized into the following 3 types: flat, depressive deformity, and bulging deformity. A multivariate logistic regression method was used to analyze associations between various data including shapes of buttonhole entry sites and occurrence of access-related infection. We also examined microscopic features of the buttonhole entry site tissue that was removed from a patient who died after 3 years of buttonhole cannulation. ***Results:*** For the flat buttonhole entry sites, frequency of access-related infection was 0.12 events/1,000 arteriovenous fistulas as compared to 0.47 events/1,000 arteriovenous fistulas for the entry sites with bulging deformity. Such infection did not occur for the entry sites with depressive deformity. The multivariate logistic regression analysis revealed a significant association between an entry site with bulging deformity and occurrence of access-related infection (odds ratio = 5.369, p = 0.0085). Furthermore, the microscopic section showed granulations beneath the skin at the buttonhole entry site and around the buttonhole tract. ***Conclusion:*** A significant association was shown between an entry site with bulging deformity and occurrence of access-related infection. The microscopic features of the buttonhole entry site of the patient on the buttonhole method for 3 years suggest that the entity of bulging deformity at the entry site is hypertrophic granulation. 

It has been reported that vascular access-related infection occurs at a higher frequency in patients on the buttonhole method than those on the rope-ladder method [1–4]. However, a reason for the higher frequency of access-related infection in patients on the buttonhole method remains to be elucidated.

Deformity of the buttonhole entry sites is frequently observed among patients cannulated by the buttonhole method for extended periods of time. Such deformity could cause higher frequency of vascular access-related infection for two reasons. One reason may be broken pieces of scabs remaining at buttonhole entry sites. In our experience, broken pieces of scabs tend to remain at buttonhole entry sites that have deformed into a raised shape. These pieces of scabs may cause access-related infection by being pushed into the buttonhole tract at the time of buttonhole cannulation. The other reason for potentially higher frequency of vascular access-related infection may be imperfect disinfection of entry sites. When a buttonhole entry site is deformed so that the periphery of the site is elevated and the central portion depressed, the central portion of the site is unlikely to be completely disinfected. Even if the central depression is not visible to the naked eye, a microscopic depression may exist at the top of the bulging entry site where an opening of the buttonhole tract exists.

Thus, the primary purpose of this study was to determine whether deformity of the entry site is one of the risk factors of access-related infection. Using a multivariate logistic regression method, we analyzed associations between different variables including shapes of buttonhole entry sites and occurrence of access-related infection. The second purpose of this study was to determine the cause of the deformity of the buttonhole entry sites, for which we also used a multivariate logistic regression method to analyze associations between various data and the shapes of buttonhole entry sites. The third purpose of this study was to examine the microscopic features of the buttonhole entry site. We examined a microscopic section of tissue from a buttonhole entry site that had been removed from a patient who died after receiving buttonhole cannulation for 3 years.

## Methods

*Patients*
We studied 166 patients using the buttonhole method at Hino Clinic in Osaka, Japan as of June 30, 2014. There were 115 males and 51 females. The age and vintage on hemodialysis was 67.3 ± 11.9 (mean ± SD) and 61.1 ± 60.0 months, respectively. The patients had been cannulated by the buttonhole method for 14.4 ± 16.0 months using the same buttonhole tracts. Vascular access was by native arteriovenous fistula (AVF) in 152

patients, arteriovenous graft in 8 patients, and superficialized artery [5] in 6 patients. The patients were dialyzed 3 times a week for 4 h each session.

Of these patients, 154 were cannulated by the buttonhole method at the entry sites on both the arterial side and venous side. However, 4 patients were cannulated only at arterial-side entry sites by the buttonhole method and 8 patients only at venous-side entry sites by the same method. Regardless of whether a buttonhole entry site was on the arterial side or on the venous side, all entry sites were analyzed together.

The etiology of kidney diseases was chronic nephritis in 37 patients, diabetic nephropathy in 77 patients, nephrosclerosis in 11 patients, polycystic kidney in 5 patients, pyelonephritis in 3 patients, other kidney diseases in 11 patients, and unknown kidney diseases in the remaining 27 patients.

*Creation of a Buttonhole Tract*
Cannulation was performed using sharp needles for 4 weeks (12 sessions) to create a buttonhole tract.

*Disinfection of Buttonhole Entry Sites and Buttonhole Cannulation*
Before hemodialysis, the buttonhole entry sites still covered by scabs were disinfected with 75% alcohol. The scabs were removed with disposable plastic tweezers to be disinfected again with a 10% povidone-iodine solution. Finally, 17-gauge dull needles (Painless Needle®, Medikit Co., Ltd., Tokyo, Japan) were inserted into each of the arterial- and venous-side buttonhole tracts.

*Statistical Analysis*
Data Analyzed
*Occurrence of Access-Related Infection.* During an 18-month period between December 30, 2012 and June 30, 2014, based on descriptions of the attending physicians, we retrieved information from the charts as to whether vascular access-related infection occurred in either arterial- or venous-side buttonhole entry sites. The physicians at our facility determine occurrence of local access-related infection in the event of the following: redness, swelling, warmth and/or presence of pus at the buttonhole entry sites, and occurrence of systemic infection originating from vascular access. However, there were no records of systemic infection in the charts during an 18-month period between December 30, 2012 and June 30, 2014.

*Shapes of Buttonhole Entry Site.* We took enlarged images of the buttonhole entry sites at ×3.7 from a distance of 18.7 mm using an enlargement camera (TG-3 Olympus®, Tokyo, Japan) after scabs were removed prior to hemodialysis. On the basis of this picture, by height of the entry site skin from the skin on the surrounding portion, we categorized shapes of buttonhole entry sites into 3 types – flat, depressive deformity, and bulging deformity (fig. 1).

*Durations from the Day When the Buttonhole Cannulation Was Started until June 30, 2014.* Information was retrieved from the chart for each patient regarding the date on which buttonhole cannulation was started for both the arterial-side and venous-side buttonhole tracts. Based on those dates, we calculated the number of months from the day when buttonhole cannulation was started until June 30, 2014.

*Durations from the Day When Hemodialysis Was Started until June 30, 2014.* From the chart of each patient, we retrieved the date of the start of hemodialysis. Based on this date, we calculated the number of years on hemodialysis until June 30, 2014.

    Sato · Shinzato · Sakai · Ohkuri · Sasaki · Nakai · Toma

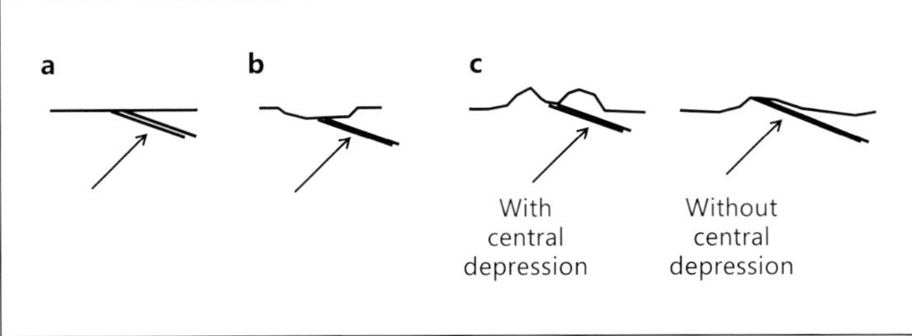

**Fig. 1.** Shapes of buttonhole entry sites: flat type (**a**), depressive deformity type (**b**), and bulging deformity type (**c**). The bulging deformity type can be further categorized into a deformity with and without a central depression visible to the naked eye on the peak. The arrows indicate buttonhole tracts.

Multivariate Analysis

*Risk of Vascular Access-Related Infection.* A multivariate logistic regression analysis was performed using occurrence of vascular access-related infection for the past 18 months as the dependent variable. The following independent variables were studied: the shape of the buttonhole entry site, number of months after the start of buttonhole cannulation, number of years after the start of hemodialysis, gender, age, vascular side of buttonhole tract (arterial side or venous side), kidney disease, and kind of vascular access (native AVF, arteriovenous graft, or superficialized artery).

*Factors for Deformation of the Buttonhole Entry Site.* The purpose of this study section was to analyze factors (by multivariate logistic regression method) that deform a flat buttonhole entry site to either a depressive deformity type or a bulging deformity type. However, when there are more than three dependent variables – a flat type, a depressive deformity type, and a bulging deformity type – a multivariate logistic regression analysis could not be performed.

The analysis was first performed using the depressive deformity type of entry site as the dependent variable in the logistic regression model incorporating only the flat type and depressive deformity type. The same analysis was next performed using the bulging deformity type of entry site as the dependent variable in the model incorporating only the flat type and bulging deformity type.

In both analyses, the independent variables were as follows: number of months after the start of buttonhole cannulation, number of years after the start of hemodialysis, gender, age, vascular side of buttonhole tract (arterial side or venous side), kidney disease, and kind of vascular access (native AVF, AVF graft, or superficialized artery).

*Microscopic Features of the Buttonhole Entry Site Tissue*
We examined microscopic features of the buttonhole entry site tissue that had been extracted from a patient who died after receiving buttonhole cannulation for 3 years. The patient was a 62-year-old male and had been on hemodialysis for 14 years and 6 months. The kidney disease was unknown, but it was not diabetic nephropathy. His cause of death was gastrointestinal bleeding associated with mesenteric artery obstruction. After the patient died and upon receiving permission from the patient's sole family member, the brother, we extracted a sample block of the buttonhole entry site,

**Table 1.** Multivariate-adjusted odds ratios and 95% CI for access-related infection

| Variables | Odds ratios | 95% CI | p |
|---|---|---|---|
| Sex (male = 1) | 0.408 | 0.084–1.986 | 0.2667 |
| Age (every 1 year) | 0.987 | 0.936–1.041 | 0.6333 |
| Years on hemodialysis (every 1 year) | 1.032 | 0.907–1.175 | 0.6296 |
| Months on buttonhole method (every 1 month) | 0.98 | 0.933–1.029 | 0.4091 |
| Diabetes (yes = 1) | 1.685 | 0.494–5.744 | 0.4042 |
| Artificial vessel vascular access (native vascular access = 1) | 0.794 | <0.001 and >999.999 | 0.9558 |
| Superficialized artery access (native vascular access = 1) | 0.351 | <0.001 and <174.481 | 0.7408 |
| Puncture site (arterial site = 1) | 1.772 | 0.549–5.716 | 0.3383 |
| Depressive entry site (flat entry site = 1) | 0.611 | 0.006–66.889 | 0.8369 |
| Bulging entry site (flat entry site = 1) | 5.369 | 1.536–18.764 | 0.0085 |
| Intercept = –3.3304 | | | |

including the AVF vessel. For microscopy, a thin slice was cut from the past formalin-fixed paraffin-embedded specimen, placed on a slide glass and stained by the Mallory-Azan method.

## Results

*Shape of Buttonhole Entry Site and Frequency of Access-Related Infection*
Of the 320 buttonhole entry sites of the 166 patients studied, 213 sites (66%) were the flat type, 17 (5.3%) were the depressive deformity type, and 90 (28.1%) were the bulging deformity type. During the 18-month period from December 30, 2012 and June 30, 2014, a total of 8 vascular access-related infections occurred among the 320 buttonhole entry sites. Of the 8 access-related infections, 3 occurred in the flat entry site, and 5 occurred in the bulging deformity type. No access-related infection occurred in the depressive deformity type.

Based on these data, the frequency of access-related infection was calculated in each shape of buttonhole entry site. The frequency of such infection was 0.12 events/1,000 AVF for the flat type and 0.47 events/1,000 AVF for the bulging deformity type.

*Risk of Vascular Access-Related Infection*
The multivariate logistic regression analysis using occurrence of vascular access-related infection for the past 18 months as the dependent variable showed that a bulging deformity of the buttonhole entry site had a significant association with access-related infection (odds ratio = 5.369, 95% CI = 1.536–18.764, p = 0.0085; table 1). There were no significant associations between vascular access-related infection and the rest of the independent variables.

**Table 2.** Multivariate-adjusted odds ratios and 95% CI for depressive buttonhole entry site deformity

| Variables | Odds ratios | 95% CI | p |
| --- | --- | --- | --- |
| Sex (male = 1) | 0.344 | 0.105–1.133 | 0.0794 |
| Age (every 1 year) | 0.967 | 0.931–1.005 | 0.0907 |
| Years on hemodialysis (every 1 year) | 1.038 | 0.933–1.155 | 0.4946 |
| Months on buttonhole method (every 1 month) | 1.092 | 1.061–1.123 | <0.0001 |
| Diabetes (yes = 1) | 1.457 | 0.571–3.723 | 0.4311 |
| Artificial vessel vascular access (native vascular access = 1) | 1.122 | 0.009–146.369 | 0.9631 |
| Superficialized artery access (native vascular access = 1) | 0.426 | 0.016–11.665 | 0.6134 |
| Puncture site (arterial site = 1) | 0.881 | 0.348–2.23 | 0.7884 |
| Intercept = –1.3909 | | | |

**Table 3.** Multivariate-adjusted odds ratios and 95% CI for bulging buttonhole entry site deformity

| Variables | Odds ratios | 95% CI | p |
| --- | --- | --- | --- |
| Sex (male = 1) | 1.093 | 0.635–1.883 | 0.7484 |
| Age (every 1 year) | 0.982 | 0.961–1.003 | 0.0851 |
| Years on hemodialysis (every 1 year) | 1.013 | 0.96–1.07 | 0.6298 |
| Months on buttonhole method (every 1 month) | 1.017 | 1.00–1.035 | 0.0562 |
| Diabetes (yes = 1) | 1.529 | 0.917–2.551 | 0.1037 |
| Artificial vessel vascular access (native vascular access = 1) | 0.276 | 0.018–4.342 | 0.3598 |
| Superficialized artery access (native vascular access = 1) | 0.238 | 0.027–2.093 | 0.1956 |
| Puncture site (arterial site = 1) | 0.843 | 0.511–1.39 | 0.5032 |
| Intercept = 0.0392 | | | |

*Factors for Deformation of Buttonhole Entry Site*

The multivariate logistic regression analysis using the depressive deformity of the entry sites as the dependent variable showed that there was a significantly association with this kind of deformity months after initiation of buttonhole cannulation (odds ratio = 1.092, 95% CI = 1.061–1.123, p < 0.0001; table 2). There were no statistically significant associations between the depressive deformity of the entry site and rest of the independent variables.

On the other hand, multivariate logistic regression analysis using the bulging deformity of the entry sites as the dependent variable showed no significant associations between this kind of deformity and any of the independent variables (table 3).

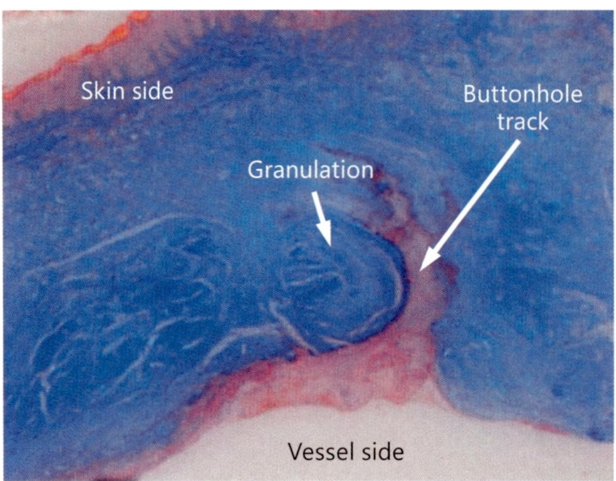


**Fig. 2.** Microscopic features of the buttonhole entry site tissue. The section was extracted from a patient who died after receiving buttonhole cannulation for 3 years. The section was stained by the Mallory-Azan method. Granulation was observed beneath the skin and in the 3- to 5-mm range from the buttonhole tract. There was also skin proliferation in the granulation area.

*Microscopic Features of the Buttonhole Entry Site Tissue*
As shown in figure 2, granulation was observed beneath the skin at the buttonhole entry site and in the 3- to 5-mm range from the buttonhole tract. There was skin proliferation in the granulation area.

## Discussion

In the present study, it was indicated that a bulging deformity of the buttonhole entry site was the only risk factor for vascular access-related infection. The access-related infection for a bulging deformity type was 5.369 times more at risk of infection than the flat type. Additionally, the frequency of access-related infection in a bulging deformity type was 0.47 events/1,000 AVF versus 0.12 events/1,000 AVF in the flat entry site. Two possible explanations can be given as the reasons for the higher frequency of the access-related infection with a bulging deformity of the buttonhole entry sites.

One reason might be incomplete removal of scabs due to the non-flat surface of the entry site. Remaining pieces of the broken scabs at the entry sites may cause access-related infection if they are pushed into the buttonhole tract when the dull needle is inserted.

The other reason might be imperfect disinfection of the buttonhole entry site. In some buttonhole entry sites with a bulging deformity, a depression has often



Sato · Shinzato · Sakai · Ohkuri · Sasaki · Nakai · Toma

been observed at the peak of a bulging deformity, as shown in figure 1. Even if such central depression is not visible to the naked eye, a microscopic depression may exist at the top of the deformity where an opening of the buttonhole tract exists. If a depression is formed at the top of the bulging deformity, rubbing the depressed central portion with a cotton ball soaked in disinfectant may not be effective and thus increases frequency of access-related infection. Nevertheless, such infection can be prevented by creating a new buttonhole tract whenever a prominent bulging deformity is formed at the buttonhole entry site.

In the present study, we examined microscopic features of buttonhole entry site tissue that had been extracted from a patient who died after receiving buttonhole cannulation for 3 years. The microscopic section showed granulation beneath the skin at the buttonhole entry site and around the buttonhole tract. Moreover, there was skin proliferation in the granulation area. These observations suggest that the entity of the bulging deformity was hypertrophic granulations that were formed under the skin of the entry site. Such hypertrophic granulation may be formed by repeated physical stimuli to the same portion of the skin.

According to a well-known theory, injury to the skin initiates a cascade of events including inflammation, fibroplasia, and contraction. If the same portion of the skin is injured repeatedly and frequently, the inflammation phase continues at the site with intensification of the degree of fibroblastic proliferation [6]. Such intensification results in excessive granulation and an increased production of scar tissue (i.e. hypertrophic granulation) [7].

In our experience, once buttonhole cannulation has been discontinued in patients with a bulging deformity of the buttonhole entry site, the deformity is resolved to normal flat skin (data not shown) in approximately 3 months. These findings support the hypothesis that hypertrophic granulation (i.e. the entity of a bulging deformity of the buttonhole entry site) is formed by repeated physical stimuli. Logically, such repeated stimulus to the skin at the entry site, by which hypertrophic granulation is formed, could be either insertion of a dull needle into the buttonhole tract or injury to the skin associated with scab removal.

In this study, we were unable to show the reasons for formation of a depressive deformity of the buttonhole entry sites. However, the entity of this type of deformity is also likely to be granulation under the skin. If the acute stage of inflammation due to skin injury associated with scab removal ends by the next hemodialysis session, the chronic stage of inflammation might not be extended, and normal remodeling of tissue develops. Thus, produced collagen is contracted so as to form the depressive deformity of the buttonhole entry sites.

These reasons for depressive deformity may be supported by the results of the present study that indicate a significant association between months after initiation of buttonhole cannulation and the depressive deformity of the entry site. A long healing period is necessary until reaching the final stage of the chronic healing process in which collagen fiber contraction occurs [8]. Therefore, a depressive deformity of the entry site will be associated with a period of time from initiation of buttonhole cannulation.

In conclusion, a significant association was indicated between frequency of access-related infection and a bulging deformity of the buttonhole entry site. The microscopic features of the buttonhole entry site of the patient on the buttonhole method for 3 years suggests that the identity of a bulging deformity of a buttonhole entry site is hypertrophic granulation.

## References


1 Gray N: The risk of sepsis from buttonhole needling must be appreciated. Nephrol Dial Transplant 2010;25:2385–2386.
2 Birchenough E, Moore C, Stevens K, et al: Buttonhole cannulation in adult patients on hemodialysis: an increased risk of infection? Nephrol Nurs J 2010;37:491–498.
3 Nesrallah GE, Cuerden M, Wong JH, et al: *Staphylococcus aureus* bacteremia and buttonhole cannulation: long-term safety and efficacy of mupirocin prophylaxis. Clin J Am Soc Nephrol 2010;5:1047–1053.
4 Labriola L, Crott R, Desmet C, et al: Infectious complications following conversion to buttonhole cannulation of native arteriovenous fistulas: a quality improvement report. Am J Kidney Dis 2011;57:442–448.
5 Sugiura S, Hata K, Funao K, et al: To preserve sources for vascular access: superficialization of radial artery at forearm. J Jpn Soc Dial Ther 2013;46:395–398.
6 McClain SA, Simon M, Jones E, et al: Mesenchymal cell activation is the rate-limiting step of granulation tissue induction. Am J Pathol 1996;149:1257–1270.
7 Fundamentals of wound healing; in Stephen Westaby (ed): Wound Care. William Heinemann Medical Books Ltd., London, 1985, pp 11–21.
8 Martin P: Wound healing – aiming for perfect skin regeneration. Science 1997;276:75–81.



Takahiro Shinzato, MD, PhD
Daiko Medical Engineering Research Institute
4-16-23 Daiko Higashi-ku Nagoya, Aichi-ken (Japan)
E-Mail shinzato@xj8.so-net.ne.jp


　Sato · Shinzato · Sakai · Ohkuri · Sasaki · Nakai · Toma

Misra M, Toma S, Shinzato T (eds): Buttonhole Cannulation: Current Prospects and Challenges.
Contrib Nephrol. Basel, Karger, 2015, vol 186, pp 57–63 (DOI: 10.1159/000431163)

# Relationship between Years Elapsed after Initial Buttonhole Cannulation and Frequency of Vascular Access-Related Infections

Shigeki Toma

Toma Clinic, Nishihara-cho, Japan

## Abstract

***Background:*** A reason for the higher frequency of vascular access-related infections in buttonhole cannulation patients remains to be elucidated. If the higher frequency of infections is associated with a factor(s) inherent to the buttonhole method (e.g. existence of a buttonhole track or other factors), the frequency of such infections is expected to increase upon starting buttonhole cannulation. On the other hand, if the higher frequency of the infections is associated with a factor(s) developing secondarily while performing buttonhole cannulation for months or years (e.g. deformity of the buttonhole entry site or other factors), the frequency is expected to rise after a certain time elapses from initiation of buttonhole cannulation. In case the higher frequency of the infections is associated with a factor(s) developing secondarily, the problem may potentially be solved. Thus, the present study is to clarify whether there is 'an infection calm period' after buttonhole cannulation is started. ***Methods:*** The relationship between the time (in years) after buttonhole cannulation is started and frequency of vascular access-related infections was investigated. ***Results:*** Frequency of access-related infections was almost constant for 6 years after buttonhole cannulation was started. At the sixth year from initiation of buttonhole cannulation, however, the frequency of access-related infections started rising. ***Conclusion:*** The rise in frequency of vascular access-related infections in buttonhole cannulation may not be directly associated with inherent factor(s) of the method, but rather a factor(s) developing secondarily while performing buttonhole cannulation over a period of years. © 2015 S. Karger AG, Basel

It has been reported that vascular-access-related infections occur at a higher frequency in buttonhole cannulation patients than in rope-ladder cannulation patients [1–4]. However, a reason for the higher frequency of infections in buttonhole cannulation patients remains to be elucidated.

The higher frequency of infections in buttonhole cannulation patients could result from not only factors inherent originally to the buttonhole method, but also to factors developing secondarily while performing buttonhole cannulation for a certain period. If the higher frequency of the access-related infections in buttonhole cannulation patients is caused by factors inherent originally to the buttonhole method (e.g. existence of buttonhole track and repeated needling at the constant site), the frequency of such infections might increase upon starting buttonhole cannulation. On the other hand, if the higher frequency of the infections is caused by a factors developing secondarily while performing buttonhole cannulation (e.g. deformity of the buttonhole entry site [5]), the frequency of infections would rise after a certain period of time elapsed from initiation of buttonhole cannulation.

Thus, the aim of the present study was to clarify the relationship between the frequency of vascular access-related infections and the period of time after initiation of buttonhole cannulation.


## Methods

*Patients*

We studied all 65 patients cannulated by the buttonhole method at the Toma Clinic as of April 1, 2014. All patients had a native arteriovenous fistula (AVF) and had been cannulated by the buttonhole method for 4.74 ± 3.94 (mean ± SD) years using the same buttonhole tracks. The patients, 36 males (age: 66.6 ± 11.69 years) and 29 females (age: 63.0 ± 12.04 years), were dialyzed 3 times a week for 4 h each session, and had been on hemodialysis for 9.84 ± 7.17 months. The etiology of kidney disease was glomerulonephritis in 42 patients, diabetes mellitus in 14 patients, nephrosclerosis in 3 patients, and other diseases in 6 patients.

*Study Design*

To clarify the relationship between the frequency of vascular access-related infections and the number of years from initiation of buttonhole cannulation, necessary data was retrieved from charts for each patient to be analyzed by the following steps.

*Step 1.* We retrieved (from the charts) the dates on which buttonhole cannulations were initiated and the dates on which vascular access-related infections occurred.

*Step 2.* We calculated, based on these data, the duration from the day when buttonhole cannulation was started until the day when a vascular access-related infection occurred for each patient who experienced such infection.

*Step 3.* We counted the number of vascular access-related infectious events for all patients in each buttonhole-cannulation year. The buttonhole-cannulation year was defined as an elapsed year from the day when the buttonhole cannulation had been started by using the buttonhole track that each patient used as of April 1, 2014.

*Step 4.* We calculated the number of patients who had been cannulated by the buttonhole method in the respective year. The calculation was based on the theory that the number of patients cannulated by the buttonhole method in the *y*th buttonhole-cannulation year (over *y – 1* years and less than *y* years from the day when the buttonhole cannulation had been started) is equivalent to the number of patients cannulated by the buttonhole method more than *y* years as of April 1, 2014.

*Step 5.* Patient-basis frequency of vascular access-related infections in any given buttonhole-cannulation year was calculated by dividing the number of access-related infectious events in this buttonhole-cannulation year by the number of patients who had been cannulated by the buttonhole method in the same year. The patient-basis frequency of vascular access-related infections was then converted to AVF day-basis frequency (i.e. vascular access-related events/1,000 AVF-days).

### *Creation of a Buttonhole Track*

At facilities in other parts of the world, cannulation was performed using sharp needles for 2 weeks (6 sessions) to create a buttonhole track [5]. In contrast, at our facility, similar to other facilities in Japan [6], cannulation was performed using a sharp needle only one time to create a buttonhole track.

### *Buttonhole Method*

Disinfectant

The buttonhole entry site was disinfected with a strong hypochlorite acid solution, which was produced on site by electrolyzing 0.1% saline at more than 1,000 mV in oxidation-reduction potential in a cell partitioned by a polyester diaphragm using an electrolyzer system (Oxilyzer®, Koken Co., Ltd., Tokyo, Japan). During electrolysis of 0.1% saline, sodium ions are attracted to the negatively charged electrodes, and chloride ions travel to the positive electrode. The chloride ions then undergo an oxidative process which results in the generation of small quantities of chlorine gas that is immediately consumed to form hydrochloric acid and hypochlorite [7].

A prepared strong hypochlorite acid solution has an acidity of 2.3–2.7 pH. Chloride ions in hypochlorite solution are in the form of HClO, ClO ion, or Cl ion, and the balance among these ions is greatly affected by the pH of the solution. In acidic pH, most of the ClO ion is in the form of HClO, and it is believed that HClO and ClO ion are effective sterilizing agents, with HClO being ten times more effective than ClO ion.

It has been reported that various bacterial strains were killed soon after being exposed to a strong hypochlorite acid solution [8–11]. Antimicrobial activity of a strong hypochlorite acid solution is similar to 80% ethanol against methicillin-sensitive *Staphylococcus aureus*, *Serratia marcescens*, *Escherichia coli*, *Pseudomonas aeruginosa*, and *Burkholderia cepacia*, but superior to 0.1% chlorhexidine and 0.02% povidone-iodine against the same bacterial strains [9].

Cannulation

Prior to disinfection of the buttonhole entry site, autonomous patients washed the access area with soap and water. Thereafter, the buttonhole entry site was disinfected using swabs soaked in a strong hypochlorite acid solution. Following disinfection, the scab created at the buttonhole entry site was removed with a sterile 18-gauge sharp needle. The site was then disinfected again using swabs soaked in strong hypochlorite acid solution. Lastly, 17-gauge dull needles (Biohole Needle®; Nipro Co., Ltd., Osaka, Japan) were inserted into the access vessel through the buttonhole track.

**Table 1.** Incidence of infectious events per period

| Duration of buttonhole cannulation, years | Patients, n | Infectious events, n |
| --- | --- | --- |
| <1 | 91 | 5 |
| >1 but <2 | 72 | 5 |
| >2 but <3 | 57 | 4 |
| >3 but <4 | 47 | 2 |
| >4 but <5 | 43 | 3 |
| >5 but <6 | 37 | 2 |
| >6 but <7 | 33 | 5 |
| >7 but <8 | 26 | 3 |
| >8 but <9 | 18 | 2 |
| >9 but <10 | 15 | 2 |
| >10 but <11 | 11 | 3 |

After hemodialysis ended, the dull needles were removed, and the site was disinfected in the same way and covered with gauze. No changes or modifications have been made to our buttonhole method for the past 10 years.

## Results

As the number of years of buttonhole cannulation progressed, the number of patients in each buttonhole-cannulation year decreased (table 1).

As shown in figure 1, the frequency of vascular access-related infections was almost constant for 5 years after initiation of buttonhole cannulation. The frequency of access-related infections was 0.34 events/1,000 AVF-days when the duration of buttonhole cannulation was <1 year, 0.44 events/1,000 AVF-days when the duration was >1 year but <2 years, 0.45 events/1,000 AVF-days when the duration was >2 years but <3 years, 0.27 events/1,000 AVF-days when the duration was >3 years but <4 years, 0.45 events/1,000 AVF-days when the duration was >4 years but <5 years, and 0.34 events/1,000 AVF-days when the duration was >5 years but <6 years. At the sixth year from initiation of buttonhole cannulation, however, the frequency of access-related infections started rising. The frequency of access-related infections was 0.97 events/1,000 AVF-days when the duration of buttonhole cannulation was >6 years but <7 years, 0.74 events/1,000 AVF-days when the duration was >7 years but <8 years, 0.71 events/1,000 AVF-days when the duration was >8 years but <9 years, 0.85 events/1,000 AVF-days when the duration was >9 years but <10 years, and 1.74 events/1,000 AVF-days when the duration was >10 years but <11 years.

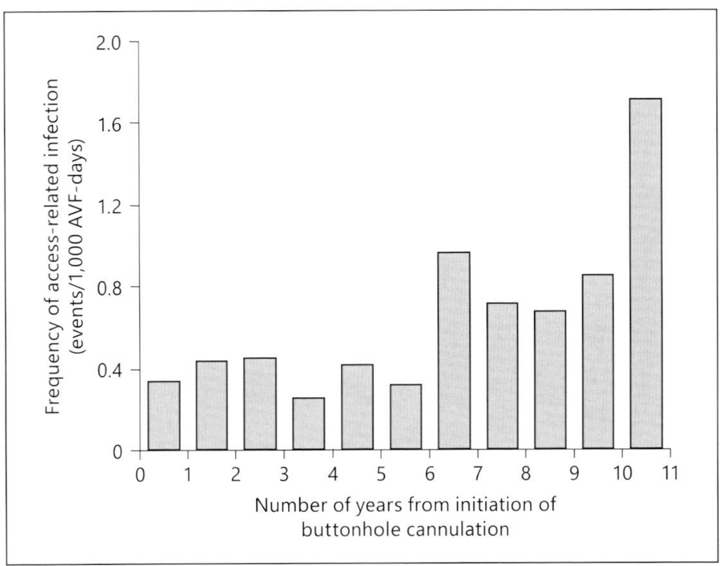


**Fig. 1.** Frequency of vascular access-related infections in each buttonhole-cannulation year. The frequency of vascular access-related infections was almost constant for 6 years after initiation of buttonhole cannulation. At the seventh year from initiation of buttonhole cannulation, however, the frequency of access-related infections started rising.

## Discussion

In the present study, it was found that there is a 6-year 'calm period' of vascular access-related infection before the frequency of infections starts to rise. These findings suggest that the rise in frequency of access-related infections in buttonhole cannulation is not directly associated with an inherent factor of the buttonhole method (e.g. existence of a buttonhole tunnel track, repeated insertion of a dull needle into the same track, or other factors), but is a factor that emerges while performing buttonhole cannulation for a certain period (e.g. deformity of the buttonhole entry site or other factors). If the rise in the frequency of infections had been directly associated with an inherent factor of the buttonhole method, the frequency would rise concurrently with the start of buttonhole cannulation.

Labriola et al. [4] showed the variation of frequency of vascular access-related infections before and after the switch from the rope-ladder method to the buttonhole method. They also showed a variation in the frequency of such infections before and after intensive staff education regarding strict protocol for the buttonhole procedure. Labriola et al. progressively replaced the rope-ladder method by the buttonhole method during the period from August 4, 2004 to

January 31, 2005, and found that the frequency of infections increased gradually between 2006 and 2007. Nevertheless, a careful review of this paper reveals that the frequency of access-related infections was rather low for almost 1 year (i.e. a calm period of vascular access-related infection) from January 31, 2005 to the end of the same year after the switch from the rope-ladder method to the buttonhole method. These data may provide evidence for the rise in frequency of access-related infections in buttonhole cannulation to be potentially associated with a secondary factor emerging while repeating cannulations at a constant site. The calm period in the patients of Labriola et al. was far shorter than in our patients. The reason is not currently known for this difference in the length of the calm period.

Sato et al. [pers. commun.] found that in some patients cannulated by the buttonhole method, the marginal portion of the buttonhole entry site becomes elevated over an extended period. Such elevation of the entry site results in a depression in the center portion where the opening of the buttonhole track exists. It may take some time for development of such a deformity. Once this deformity becomes pronounced, however, disinfection of the sunken center of the buttonhole entry site might become difficult and cause a rise in frequency of access-related infection.

In conclusion, the rise in frequency of access-related infections in buttonhole cannulation may not be directly associated with an inherent factor of the method (e.g. existence of a buttonhole tunnel track, repeated insertion of a dull needle into the same track, or other factors), but it is a factor that emerges while repeating cannulations at a constant site (e.g. deformity of the buttonhole entry site or other factors).

## References


1 Gray N: The risk of sepsis from buttonhole needling must be appreciated. Nephrol Dial Transplant 2010;25:2385–2386.
2 Birchenough E, Moore C, Stevens K, Stewart S: Buttonhole cannulation in adult patients on hemodialysis: an increased risk of infection? Nephrol Nurs J 2010;37:491–498.
3 Nesrallah GE, Cuerden M, Wong JH, Pierratos A: *Staphylococcus aureus* bacteremia and buttonhole cannulation: long-term safety and efficacy of mupirocin prophylaxis. Clin J Am Soc Nephrol 2010;5:1047–1053.
4 Labriola L, Crott R, Desmet C, André G, Jadoul M: Infectious complications following conversion to buttonhole cannulation of native arteriovenous fistulas: a quality improvement report. Am J Kidney Dis 2011;57:442–448.
5 Twardowski Z: Different sites versus constant sites of needle insertion into arteriovenous fistulas for treatment by repeated dialysis. Dial Transplant 1979;8:978–980.
6 Ogawa C, Okada K, Iijima S, Mizumori K, Otsuka K: The buttonhole method using single needling (in Japanese). J Jpn Soc Dial Ther 2010;43:989–992.

7  Kraft A, Stadelmann M, Blaschke M, Kreysig D, Sandt B, Schröder F, Rennau J: Electrochemical water disinfection part I: hypochlorite production from very dilute chloride solutions. J Appl Electrochem 1999;29:861–868.

8  Tanaka N, Fujisawa T, Daimon T, Fujiwara K, Yamamoto M, Abe T: The cleaning and disinfecting of hemodialysis equipment using electrolyzed strong acid aqueous solution. Artif Organs 1999;23:303–309.

9  Iwasawa A, Nakamura Y: Bactericidal effect of acidic electrolyzed water – comparison of chemical acidic sodium hydrochloride (NaOCl) solution (in Japanese). Kansenshogaku Zasshi 1996;70:915–922.

10  Tanaka H, Hirakata Y, Kaku M, Yoshida R, Takemura H, Mizukane R, Ishida K, Tomono K, Koga H, Kohno S, Kamihira S: Antimicrobial activity of superoxidized water. J Hosp Infect 1996;34:43–49.

11  Selkon JB, Babb R, Morris R: Evaluation of the antimicrobial activity of a new super-oxidized water, Sterilox, for the disinfection of endoscopes. J Hosp Infec 1999;41:59–70.

Shigeki Toma, MD
Toma Clinic
972 Aza-Kochi, Nishihara-cho, Nakagami-gun
Okinawa Prefecture (Japan)
E-Mail stoma@air.linkclub.or.jp

Misra M, Toma S, Shinzato T (eds): Buttonhole Cannulation: Current Prospects and Challenges.
Contrib Nephrol. Basel, Karger, 2015, vol 186, pp 64–70 (DOI: 10.1159/000431162)

# Long-Term Safety of Buttonhole Cannulation and Efficacy of Mupirocin Prophylaxis

Arnav Agarwal[a] · Gihad Nesrallah[b, c]

[a]Faculty of Medicine, University of Toronto, [b]Nephrology Program, Humber River Hospital,
and [c]The Li Ka Shing Knowledge Institute, Keenan Research Centre, St. Michael's Hospital,
Toronto, Ont., Canada

## Abstract

Buttonhole cannulation has drawn considerable interest in recent years, particularly with
the proliferation of home hemodialysis. Touted benefits of this cannulation method include reduced pain, ease of use, reduced aneurysm formation, and overall greater patient
satisfaction. However, recent studies have also suggested that systemic and local infection
rates are higher with buttonhole cannulation compared with the standard rope-ladder
method. In this review, we summarize recent systematic review findings and practice
guidelines addressing the benefits and harms of buttonhole cannulation, and discuss the
role of topical antimicrobial prophylaxis. © 2015 S. Karger AG, Basel

Arteriovenous fistulae (AVF) are associated with fewer infections and better
survival compared with catheters, and thus remain the preferred access for most
patients receiving hemodialysis [1]. Despite better long-term outcomes, AVF
use is fraught with challenges for both home and in-center hemodialysis patients
and providers. While anatomical and other clinical factors are largely not mod-
ifiable or within the provider's control, the approach to cannulation might rep-
resent a useful target for intervention for improving AVF outcomes.

Three cannulation methods have evolved over time. The area cannulation
method, which has been associated with rapid development of aneurysms and
access loss [2], has largely been abandoned in favor of the 'rope-ladder' or 'ro-
tating-site' cannulation method. With this approach, sharp-needle venipuncture is performed at new sites at each dialysis session. Though it is currently the

most widely used cannulation method, pain, needle aversion, technical complexity, and long-term patency remain significant barriers to long-term AVF use and to self-cannulation by home dialysis patients.

The buttonhole cannulation or constant-site needling technique was introduced in the 1970s for cannulation of short fistula segments [3, 4]. Buttonhole cannulation involves repeated punctures with blunt needles through established venous scar tissue tunnel tracts via the same insertion site, at the same angle, ideally by the same cannulator. A sharp needle is initially introduced into the same site over 6–9 hemodialysis sessions until a tunnel tract forms.

Buttonhole cannulation is perceived to reduce problematic cannulation episodes, patient discomfort, and access failure, and may simplify self-cannulation – an important facilitator of home dialysis. These purported benefits have led to a resurgence of the technique, and these are reviewed in other chapters in this series. Despite many potential advantages, more recent reports have suggested that buttonhole cannulation may lead to increased systemic and local infections. In this narrative review, we explore the incidence of infection with buttonhole cannulation, risk factors for infection, and potential strategies to mitigate long-term infection risks with this cannulation approach. We then review recent clinical practice recommendations and highlight priorities for future research.

## Incidence of Infection with Buttonhole Cannulation

Rates of infection and other complications with buttonhole cannulation have been reviewed extensively, with recent meta-analyses published on home and in-center hemodialysis populations [5–7]. The Canadian Society of Nephrology also conducted a systematic review of vascular access outcomes with intensive hemodialysis [8] to inform a clinical practice guideline addressing the clinical management of this unique population [9]. Several factors lower our overall confidence in reported treatment effects in individual studies comparing buttonhole with rope-ladder cannulation. These include small study sample sizes and predominantly observational designs with the usual limitations of residual confounding and selection bias. Moreover, systematic reviews and meta-analyses of these studies are limited by heterogeneity in study design and populations, which often precludes the calculation of reliable pooled treatment effect estimates.

These limitations notwithstanding, there appears to be an emerging consensus that buttonhole cannulation is associated with an increased risk of local and systemic infection. Studies that have reported on the microbiology of buttonhole cannulation-related infections have identified *Staphylococcus aureus* as a common pathogen [10–12]. Given the relatively serious nature of *S. aureus* bacteremia, this has been a matter of significant concern, with reports of septic arthritis, septic pulmonary embolism, epidural abscess, endocarditis, and even death in patients using buttonhole cannulation [10–12].

In a recent systematic review, we reported the range of bacteremia rates in patients receiving in-center hemodialysis to be 0.00–0.31 per 1,000 AVF days in 543 patients experiencing 87 events during 1,034 patient-years [5]. An informative study by Labriola and Jadoul [10] described a baseline bacteremia rate of 0.43 events per 1,000 AVF days after converting an in-center dialysis program to buttonhole cannulation. After retraining nursing staff, the infection rate fell to 0.34 events per 1,000 AVF days, suggesting that operator vigilance and technique are important predictors of infection risk. Bacteremia rates among home dialysis patients have historically ranged from 0.00 to 0.28 per 1,000 AVF days when combining results from six studies that included 416 patients followed for 1,069 patient-years. In the absence of parallel control groups in the included studies, one can contrast these rates with infection rates associated with hemodialysis catheter use in the United States and Canada, which are at 0.50 and 1.30 per 1,000 AVF days, respectively [13, 14].

In a recent meta-analysis, Muir et al. [6] reported a threefold increase in bacteremia when pooling 4 clinical trials comparing buttonhole cannulation with rope-ladder cannulation, with a pooled relative risk of 3.34 (95% CI: 0.91–12.20; $I^2 = 15\%$). This was similar in magnitude to the pooled estimate based on 8 observational studies with a relative risk of 3.27 (95% CI: 1.44–7.43; $I^2 = 0$), and also comparable to their single-center experience of 90 patients followed over 3,765 months. More recently, Wong et al. [7] conducted a similar review, but concluded that heterogeneity of case definition of infectious complications precluded meaningful pooling of infection rates. They also noted that clinical trials conducted to date were not powered to evaluate differences in infection rates, and that infection was usually a secondary outcome.

## Modifiable Practices Associated with Infection Risk in Buttonhole Cannulation

### *Patient and Provider Factors*

We recently attempted to identify patient and provider level factors associated with bacteremia rates in a systematic review of studies comparing buttonhole with rope-ladder cannulation [5]. We considered variables such as dialysis frequency, single versus multiple cannulators while establishing buttonhole tracts, single versus multiple cannulators during routine cannulation, site care protocols, native tissue buttonholes with scabs versus polycarbonate pegs, scab removal technique, use of sharp versus dull needles, and type of cannulator (lay caregiver vs. nurse) to be of potential significance; however, a small number of included studies and significant clinical heterogeneity precluded any meaningful quantitative analysis.

*Antimicrobial Prophylaxis*

We have previously described our single-center experience with topical mupirocin prophylaxis for patients undergoing home hemodialysis with AVF using buttonhole cannulation [11]. In a crossover observational study, we described rates of *S. aureus* bacteremia among 56 consecutive patients receiving home nocturnal hemodialysis. Prior to adopting a topical mupirocin prophylaxis regimen, we observed 10 episodes of bacteremia, with metastatic complications in 4 cases. We subsequently introduced topical mupirocin prophylaxis with mupirocin applied with a cotton swab applicator to buttonhole sites after decannulation and hemostasis. Following this intervention we observed two additional episodes of bacteremia during follow-up, but only among patients who did not adhere to the prescribed mupirocin regimen. Using logistic regression, the odds ratio for *S. aureus* bacteremia was 35.3 (95% CI: 2.0–626.7; p = 0.01) for patients not using mupirocin.

## Current Practice Guidelines

Practice guidelines addressing aspects of buttonhole cannulation are few, and largely consist of informal guidance published as narrative reviews based on expert opinion. In 2013, the Canadian Society of Nephrology published a practice guideline that included recommendations for vascular access management for patients undergoing intensive (longer or more frequent than conventional) hemodialysis. The guideline was not intended to address similar management questions for in-center conventional dialysis recipients.

The guideline was developed using the Grading of Recommendations Assessment, Development and Evaluation (GRADE) framework. In the GRADE approach, guideline developers identify and prioritize clinical management questions (framed as 'population', 'intervention', 'comparator', and 'outcome' – 'PICO' questions) with a focus on patient-important outcomes, then perform systematic reviews and meta-analyses addressing these questions [15]. The quality of evidence for each question is rated across 5 domains (imprecision, inconsistency, risk of bias, indirectness, and publication bias), resulting in an overall quality rating [16]. Quality ratings range from very low to high, and denote the overall confidence in each estimate of effect [17]. Guideline developers can then consider the quality of evidence, economic factors, and patient values and preferences when issuing a recommendation. Strong recommendations are usually based on moderate-to-high quality evidence, and/or when on balance it is expected that the recommended course of action will cause significant benefit with minimal harm in a majority of cases. When there is greater uncertainty around the effectiveness of an intervention, guideline developers will typically issue a weak or conditional recommendation, in which providers are encouraged to engage patients in shared decision making, highlighting the risks and benefits of the alternative treatment approaches, and helping patients to incorporate their values and preferences into the decision-making process.

The CSN Intensive Hemodialysis Guideline included three recommendations related to vascular access practices, including choice of access type, choice of cannulation method, and the use of topical mupirocin for preventing infection in patients using buttonhole cannulation [9].

The panel issued a conditional recommendation favoring the use of arteriovenous access over catheters [9]. In formulating this recommendation, the panel considered the harm associated with a potentially higher infection rate with catheters to outweigh any potential benefits such as avoidance of sharp-needle cannulation or shorter training time for home dialysis that might be conferred by catheters. The recommendation was conditional due to very low-quality evidence, with no randomized trials and reliance on observational studies with a high risk of bias due to limited case-mix adjustment, selection bias, and other factors.

For patients using AVF, the panel addressed the cannulation approach as follows: 'For adult end-stage renal disease patients receiving intensive home hemodialysis with an AV fistula, we suggest the use of rope-ladder cannulation over buttonhole cannulation, unless topical antimicrobial prophylaxis is used' [9]. This recommendation placed a higher value on preventing systemic infections over avoiding repeated sharp-needle cannulation and potentially shorter home hemodialysis training times conferred by buttonhole cannulation. The panel acknowledged that the overall quality of evidence informing this recommendation was very low, again due to a reliance on observational studies. The panel also recommended full disclosure to patients of potential risks of buttonhole cannulation, and recommended obtaining written informed consent from patients [9]. The panel also acknowledged the role for buttonhole cannulation for patients with short usable segments, aneurysms, or other unique anatomical considerations that precluded routine rope-ladder cannulation.

Finally, the panel issued the following guidance for the use of mupirocin prophylaxis for buttonhole cannulation: 'For adult end-stage renal disease patients using buttonhole cannulation for intensive home hemodialysis, we suggest the use of mupirocin antibacterial cream to reduce the risk of infection' [9]. This recommendation prioritized infection prevention over the theoretical risk of mupirocin resistance, patient inconvenience with cream application, and cost of the cream. The recommendation was also conditional and based on very low-quality evidence, with only one pre-post study available to compare benefits and harms.

In 2006, the KDOQI Vascular Access guidelines suggested that buttonhole cannulation could be considered for patients who self-cannulate, and for patients with AVF in general [18]. The recommendation was ungraded, and was based on then recent studies suggesting less cannulation pain, greater ease of self-cannulation, and less frequent infiltration. More recently, however, since there have been concerns related to infection risk and lack of compelling evidence of other benefits such as reduced pain with cannulation [19], we would generally not advocate for routine buttonhole cannulation in unselected in-center hemodialysis populations until higher-quality evidence of safety and efficacy becomes available [20]. Where it is routinely provided to in-center patients, it would seem reasonable to carefully track infection rates, and to ensure ongoing staff training, competency, and vigilance. Using buttonhole cannulation to restore the function of an aneurysmal or anatomically challenging fistula has been reported and might be considered for use in these selected cases [21]. However, even with careful and restricted use of the technique, infections have been reported [22].

## Implications for Future Research

The literature describing optimal vascular access practices remains controversial and is largely based on observational studies with significant methodological limitations. Better confidence in measures of infection risk with available cannulation methods is needed, as is a better understanding of the comparative effects on long-term patency and patient-reported outcomes such as comfort and ease of use.

Many have called for randomized trials comparing cannulation methods [12, 20, 23], yet the renal community also recognizes the many logistical issues that thwart large clinical trials, including frequent patient attrition, small and dispersed populations requiring multicentered designs, patient willingness, and costs, to name a few. These challenges call for more innovative approaches to research design – preference-based randomized trials, cluster-randomized and registry-based trials, and rigorous prospective observational studies seem worthy of further exploration. Until new research approaches lead to higher-quality and more feasible studies, considerable uncertainty will continue to surround important aspects of dialysis practice, including vascular access management.

## References

1 Lok CE, Foley R: Vascular access morbidity and mortality: trends of the last decade. Clin J Am Soc Nephrol 2013;8:1213–1219.

2 Parisotto MT, Schoder VU, Miriunis C, et al: Cannulation technique influences arteriovenous fistula and graft survival. Kidney Int 2014;86:790–797.

3 Twardowski Z, Lebek R, Kubara H: 6-year experience with the creation and use of internal arteriovenous fistulae in patients treated with repeated hemodialysis (in Polish). Pol Arch Med Wewn 1977;57:205–214.

4 Twardowski Z: Different sites versus constant sites of needle insertion into arteriovenous fistulas for treatment of repeated dialysis. Dial Transplant 1979;8:978–980.

5 Grudzinski A, Mendelssohn D, Pierratos A, et al: A systematic review of buttonhole cannulation practices and outcomes. Semin Dial 2013;26:465–475.

6 Muir CA, Kotwal SS, Hawley CM, et al: Buttonhole cannulation and clinical outcomes in a home hemodialysis cohort and systematic review. Clin J Am Soc Nephrol 2014;9:110–119.

7 Wong B, Muneer M, Wiebe N, et al: Buttonhole versus rope-ladder cannulation of arteriovenous fistulas for hemodialysis: a systematic review. Am J Kidney Dis 2014;64:918–936.

8 Mustafa RA, Zimmerman D, Rioux JP, et al: Vascular access for intensive maintenance hemodialysis: a systematic review for a Canadian Society of Nephrology clinical practice guideline. Am J Kidney Dis 2013;62:112–131.

9 Nesrallah GE, Mustafa RA, Macrae J, et al: Canadian Society of Nephrology guidelines for the management of patients with ESRD treated with intensive hemodialysis. Am J Kidney Dis 2013;62:187–198.

10 Labriola L, Jadoul M: Infectious complications following conversion to buttonhole cannulation. Clin Nephrol 2011;76:423, author reply 424.

11 Nesrallah GE, Cuerden M, Wong JH, et al: *Staphylococcus aureus* bacteremia and buttonhole cannulation: long-term safety and efficacy of mupirocin prophylaxis. Clin J Am Soc Nephrol 2010;5:1047–1053.

12 Lok CE, Sontrop JM, Faratro R, et al: Frequent hemodialysis fistula infectious complications. Nephron Extra 2014;4:159–167.

13 Taylor G, Gravel D, Johnston L, et al: Incidence of bloodstream infection in multicenter inception cohorts of hemodialysis patients. Am J Infect Control 2004;32:155–160.

14 Dryden MS, Samson A, Ludlam HA, et al: Infective complications associated with the use of the Quinton 'Permcath' for long-term central vascular access in haemodialysis. J Hosp Infect 1991;19:257–262.

15 Guyatt GH, Oxman AD, Kunz R, et al: GRADE guidelines: 2. Framing the question and deciding on important outcomes. J Clin Epidemiol 2011;64:395–400.

16 Guyatt G, Oxman AD, Akl EA, et al: GRADE guidelines: 1. Introduction – GRADE evidence profiles and summary of findings tables. J Clin Epidemiol 2011;64:383–394.

17 Balshem H, Helfand M, Schunemann HJ, et al: GRADE guidelines: 3. Rating the quality of evidence. J Clin Epidemiol 2011;64:401–406.

18 Vascular Access Work Group: Clinical practice guidelines for vascular access. Am J Kidney Dis 2006;48(suppl 1):S248–S273.

19 Macrae JM, Ahmed SB, Atkar R, et al: A randomized trial comparing buttonhole with rope ladder needling in conventional hemodialysis patients. Clin J Am Soc Nephrol 2012;7:1632–1638.

20 Moist LM, Nesrallah GE: Should buttonhole cannulation be discontinued? Clin J Am Soc Nephrol 2014;9:3–5.

21 Marticorena RM, Hunter J, Macleod S, et al: The salvage of aneurysmal fistulae utilizing a modified buttonhole cannulation technique and multiple cannulators. Hemodial Int 2006;10:193–200.

22 van Loon MM, Goovaerts T, Kessels AG, et al: Buttonhole needling of haemodialysis arteriovenous fistulae results in less complications and interventions compared to the rope-ladder technique. Nephrol Dial Transplant 2010;25:225–230.

23 Atkar RK, MacRae JM: The buttonhole technique for fistula cannulation: pros and cons. Curr Opin Nephrol Hypertens 2013;22:629–636.

Gihad Nesrallah, MD, MSc, FRCPC
The Li Ka Shing Knowledge Institute
Keenan Research Centre, St. Michael's Hospital
30 Bond Street, Toronto, ON M5B 1W8 (Canada)
E-Mail gnesrallah@hrh.ca

Misra M, Toma S, Shinzato T (eds): Buttonhole Cannulation: Current Prospects and Challenges.
Contrib Nephrol. Basel, Karger, 2015, vol 186, pp 71–78 (DOI: 10.1159/000431167)

# Application of Buttonhole Cannulation Technique to Surgically Superficialized Arteries

Kunihiro Hayakawa[a] · Daiki Sugiyama[a] · Hiroaki Tanaka[a] ·
Satoshi Shinohara[c] · Takahiro Ohki[b] · Akinori Muraoka[b] ·
Masamiki Miwa[d]

[a]Satsukinomori Clinic, Hamamatsu, [b]Atsumi Medical Clinic, Tahara, and [c]Ohzone Clinic, and
[d]Atsuta Clinic, Nagoya, Japan

**Abstract**

In Japan, use of a surgically superficialized brachial artery is recommended for vascular access in patients who are either unable to tolerate hemodialysis because of reduced cardiac function or who do not have vessels suitable for creation of an arteriovenous fistula. Superficializing a brachial artery involves relocating a portion of the artery into subcutaneous tissue and immobilizing the artery at that location. Superficialized artery access can result in certain serious complications, such as an aneurysm and/or stenosis. In order to avoid such complications, we attempted applying the buttonhole method to this vascular access. A buttonhole track was created slightly distal from the center of the superficialized portion of a brachial artery approximately 2 weeks after superficialization. When arteriosclerosis was evident in that location, we tried to find a less sclerotic portion, under ultrasonography guidance, for creation of the arterial-side buttonhole track. For returning extracorporeal circulated blood, a normal vein on the arm with a superficialized brachial artery was cannulated with a sharp needle. Recently, however, we attempted to create a buttonhole track also on a vein for venous-side buttonhole cannulation. The brachial artery was superficialized in 5 patients. In all patients, buttonhole cannulation was successfully performed with the artery access. Buttonhole cannulation had been performed on these patients for 8–54 months. No serious complications such as a pseudoaneurysm were found in these patients. Serious complications specific to the superficialized artery access may be prevented by application of the buttonhole method.                    © 2015 S. Karger AG, Basel

In recent years, the patient population with severe arteriosclerosis, heart failure, and/or diabetes mellitus has increased. Such patients tend not to be able to tolerate hemodialysis treatment. In these kinds of patients in Japan, use of a surgically superficialized brachial artery for vascular access is recommended [1, 2].

A major drawback of this new vascular access is the ease of aneurysm and/or stenosis formation [3] due to limited puncture locations. One potential option may be the buttonhole method [4–7].

In this article, we will first describe the method of formation of superficialized brachial artery access in addition to its advantages and disadvantages. We will next indicate the results of the buttonhole method application to this vascular access.

## Superficialization of a Deep Artery

*Superficialized Femoral Artery Access and Brachial Artery Access*
Superficialized artery access was first reported by Brittinger et al. [8] in 1970. They superficialized a portion of a femoral artery for use as vascular access. However, superficialized femoral artery access had a number of disadvantages.

A wide operation field is required to superficialize a portion of a femoral artery, and therefore formation of the superficialized femoral artery access requires general or spinal anesthesia. A subcutaneous pocket created to hold the superficialized portion of the femoral artery has often been observed to fill with lymphatic fluid exuding from the lining of the pocket. It has also been reported that necrosis of the sutured part of the skin has occasionally occurred [9]. Due to such complications relating to superficialized femoral artery access, in Japan the superficialized brachial artery access is formed in almost all cases under local anesthesia [10].

*Current Status of Superficialized Brachial Artery Access*
Based on a report of the Statistical Survey Committee of the Japanese Society for Dialysis Therapy, superficialized brachial artery access was used in 3,146 (1.8%) patients among 172,244 patients surveyed [11]. Murotani et al. [12] reported that the reason for selection of superficialized brachial artery access was reduced cardiac function in 73% of their patients, lack of an appropriate vein for creation of arteriovenous fistula (AVF) in 19% of the patients, and miscellaneous in the remaining 8% of the patients.

     

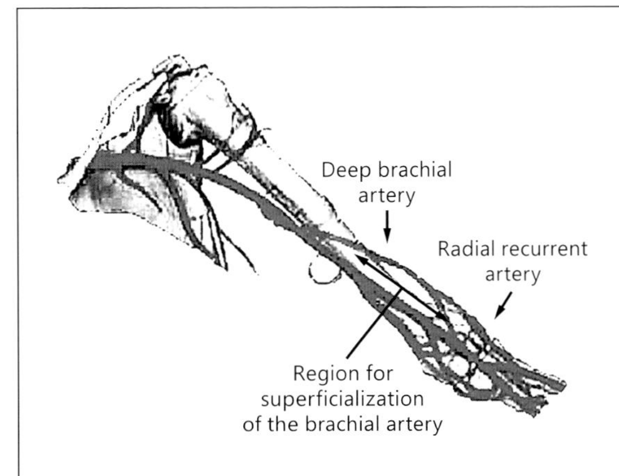


**Fig. 1.** Collateral vessels of the brachial artery. In the upper arm, the radial recurrent artery serves as a collateral vessel of the brachial artery.

*Indications for Superficialized Brachial Artery Access*

The Japanese Society for Dialysis Therapy provides indications for superficialized brachial artery access as follows:

(1) Cases in which cardiac overload due to the presence of an AVF is not tolerated (cases in which cardiac ejection fraction is less than 30% by echocardiogram)

(2) Cases in which creation of an AVF is difficult because of thin native veins

(3) Cases in which steal syndrome is predicted to develop if an AVF is created, or steal syndrome has already developed due to existence of an AVF

(4) Cases in which venous hypertension is predicted to develop if an AVF is created, or venous hypertension has already developed due to existence of an AVF

(5) Cases in which alternative vascular access is necessary because of frequent difficulties of AVF vessel puncture [13]

*Procedure to Superficialize a Brachial Artery*

*Presence of a Puncturable Subcutaneous Vein.* Prior to surgery, it needs to be determined whether a puncturable subcutaneous vein for returning extracorporeal circulating blood is present in the arm in which the brachial artery is to be superficialized. We regard a vein large enough to be used for regular blood sampling as a real puncturable vein. In case of the absence of a vein to meet such criteria, superficialized brachial artery access may not be formed.

*Collateral Vessels of the Brachial Artery.* In the upper arm, as shown in figure 1, the radial recurrent artery serves as a collateral vessel of the brachial artery. In the worst case scenario of superficialized brachial artery obstruction, blood flow in this collateral vessel prevents peripheral ischemia. Therefore, prior to surgery,

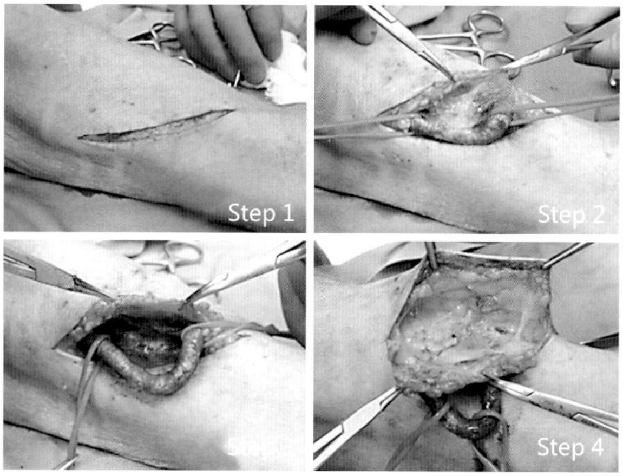

**Fig. 2.** Process of the first half of the operation. Step 1: skin incision, step 2: incision of the fascia, step 3: exposure of the brachial artery, and step 4: creation of the subcutaneous pocket.

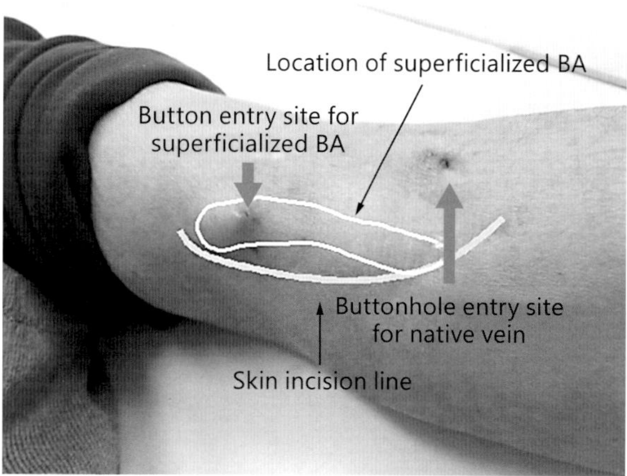


**Fig. 3.** Locations of skin incision for operation, superficialized portion of the brachial artery, and buttonhole entry sites for the superficialized brachial artery (BA) and the native vein.

it must be determined whether the radial recurrent artery is not occluded in the arm in which the brachial artery is to be superficialized.

*Surgical Procedure.* The process of the first half of the operation is shown in steps 1–4 in figure 2. An approximate 12-cm incision is made into the skin medially between 2 and 3 cm (fig. 3) from the brachial artery (step 1). Following the fascia incision (step 2), a cubital-side portion of the brachial artery is exposed at a length approximately one third of the upper arm (step 3; fig. 3). Thereafter, the skin above the brachial artery is detached to create a space for the superficialized portion of the brachial artery, i.e. a subcutaneous pocket (step 4). When the skin is detached, an appropriate amount of adipose tissue must remain on the skin. The amount of adipose tissue remaining on the skin determines the depth of the superficialized brachial artery. Brachial artery access that is too deep will



Hayakawa · Sugiyama · Tanaka · Shinohara · Ohki · Muraoka · Miwa

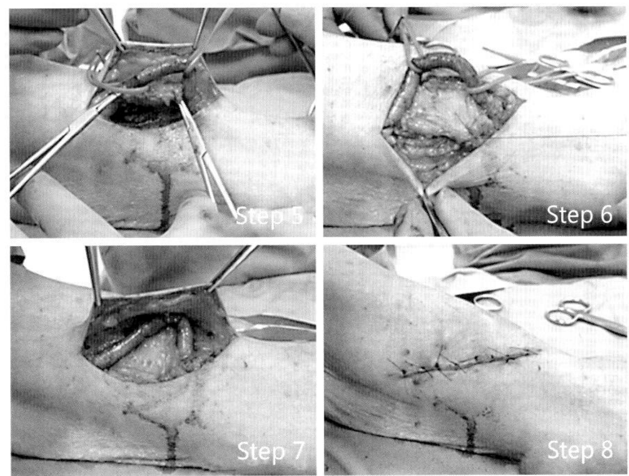


**Fig. 4.** Process of the second half of the operation. Step 5: placement of the stumps of the incised fascia beneath the exposed brachial artery, step 6: suture of the stumps of the incised fascia, step 7: immobilization of the superficialized brachial artery, and step 8: suture of the incised skin.

cause difficulties in needling, and it being too shallow will cause necrosis of a suture part of the skin and also prolong hemostasis time.

The process of the second half of the operation is shown from step 5 through step 8 in figure 4. The stumps of the incised fascia are sutured to each other under the brachial artery that is exposed for superficialization (steps 5 and 6), followed by immobilization of the superficialized brachial artery in the subcutaneous tissue with several stiches (step 7). Finally, the incised portion of the skin is closed to complete the surgical procedure (step 8).

### Cannulation of a Superficialized Brachial Artery

Prior to cannulation of the superficialized brachial artery, a puncture site on the skin is disinfected with 10% povidone-iodine solution. At every hemodialysis session, the superficialized brachial artery is cannulated with a 17-gauge sharp needle at a different site in a relatively narrow segment (8–10 cm) that is allowed for cannulation. In patients with severe arteriosclerosis, the allowed segment for cannulation is often much narrower due to calcification of vascular walls.

For venous-side cannulation, a normal vein on the arm with a superficialized brachial artery is cannulated also with a 17-gauge sharp needle at a different site in a wide range.

### Hemostasis

At the time hemodialysis is completed, pressure is applied to the entry site by one's index finger with enough strength that the arterial pulse can be felt. During the procedure, close attention should be paid not to stop blood flow through the brachial artery.

*Complications*

Complications shortly after surgery include bleeding, formation of hematomas, and lymphorrhea, whereas late complications include infection, obstruction, and arterial dilation, i.e. an aneurysm.

An aneurysm is categorized as either a true aneurysm or a pseudoaneurysm. A true aneurysm is a fusiform arterial expansion maintaining a perfect three-layer arterial wall structure. A pseudoaneurysm, in contrast, is a partial expansion of the arterial wall with disruption of the normal three-layer structure.

In our experience, as well as a report by Hamada et al. [13], true aneurysms were observed in almost all cases in which superficialized brachial artery access had been used for over 12 months. Risk of rupture is minimal for true aneurysms, which still require close monitoring of further development while continuing use. In case of a pseudoaneurysm, however, early surgical treatment is necessary due to a high risk of rupture.

## Application of the Buttonhole Method to Superficialized Brachial Artery Access

Patients for whom creation of superficialized brachial artery access has been decided usually have no alternative vessels for vascular access. Therefore, complications of pseudoaneurysms and stenosis are more serious for patients with a superficialized brachial artery than those with an AVF. Nevertheless, these complications are more frequent with a superficialized brachial artery than an AVF because superficialized brachial artery access is characterized by high pressure and limited possible locations for cannulation.

These complications of superficialized brachial artery access are potentially prevented by buttonhole cannulation. Moreover, when buttonhole cannulation is applied to superficialized brachial artery access, incidence of the trampoline effect, which often occurs for AVF, decreases greatly. Such advantages indicate the most appropriate cannulation method is the buttonhole method with superficialized brachial artery access.

*Creation of Buttonhole Tracks*

Even for a superficialized brachial artery, buttonhole tracks are created using the same method as in normal AVF. Approximately 2 weeks after brachial artery superficialization surgery, buttonhole tracks are created by cannulating the same site of the artery by a sharp needle over six consecutive sessions during a 2-week period.

For the reason of easy application of pressure by one's finger for hemostasis, as a fundamental rule, a buttonhole track is created at a location slightly distal

  Hayakawa · Sugiyama · Tanaka · Shinohara · Ohki · Muraoka · Miwa from the center of the superficialized portion of the artery (fig. 2). In the event that there is a marked atheroma at that site, a buttonhole track is created under ultrasonography guidance at a site slightly apart from the original site.

In the upper arm with a superficialized brachial artery, in the event that there is only one appropriate vein to which extracorporeal circulating blood returns, we create buttonhole tracks in the vein to prolong the life of the vessel as a vascular access site (fig. 3).

Buttonhole tracks to veins are created with the same method as buttonhole tracks to AVF. In our experience, it appears that cannulation by the buttonhole method prolongs vein life more than the rope-ladder method.

### Disinfection and Buttonhole Cannulation

There is no difference in the buttonhole method between superficialized brachial artery access and AVF. Prior to starting hemodialysis, the buttonhole entry site with a scab is disinfected by using a 75% alcohol solution before the scab is removed. After the scab is removed, the site is disinfected again using a 10% povidone-iodine solution.

Thereafter, a superficialized brachial artery is cannulated with a 17-gauge needle (Dull AVF Needle; Nipro Co., Ltd., Osaka, Japan) through the buttonhole track. Even with the vein, disinfection and buttonhole cannulation are performed by the same method.

### Hemostasis

After removal of a dull needle when completing hemodialysis, any bleeding is stopped by applying pressure for 15 min to the entry site with one's index finger. During the hemostatic procedure, appropriate pressure should be applied to the entry site to allow the arterial pulse to be felt without stopping blood flow through the superficialized brachial artery.

Currently, we apply pressure to the entry site for another 20 min using a pressure bandage to ensure that recurrent bleeding does not occur after patients leave our facility. Extended pressure application to a superficialized brachial artery, however, could cause thrombus formation. From the viewpoint of such a risk, whether additional pressure should be applied is a topic for future consideration.

## Conclusions

Superficialized brachial artery access is one solution for patients with severely reduced cardiac function and those for which AVF creation is difficult. Nevertheless, this vascular access also has serious complications (e.g. an aneurysm and stenosis). A combination of this vascular access and buttonhole cannulation, however, potentially reduces such complications.

Combining superficialized brachial artery access with the buttonhole method could potentially be indicated even for patients who do not have any reduced cardiac function. This combined approach could thus prevent such cardiac diseases from developing in the future.

## References


1 Ohira S, Naito H, Amano I, et al: 2005 Japanese Society for Dialysis Therapy guidelines for vascular access construction and repair for chronic hemodialysis. Ther Apher Dial 2006;10:449–462.

2 Gouya T: Superficialized artery; in Gouya T (ed): Standard Blood Access (in Japanese). Tokyo, Shindan to Chiryou-sha, 1999, pp 59–62.

3 Matsuo K, Yasunaga N, Nakamoto M, et al: The results and complications of superficialized artery access (in Japanese). Kidney Dial 2001, pp 33–35.

4 Twardowski Z: Different sites versus constant sites of needle insertion into arteriovenous fistulas for treatment by repeated dialysis. Dial Transplant 1979;8:978–980.

5 Scribner BH: Circulatory access: still a major concern. Proc Eur Dial Transplant Assoc 1982;19:95–98.

6 Scribner BH: The overriding importance of vascular access. Dial Transplant 1984;13:635–638.

7 Twardowski Z: Constant site (buttonhole) method of needle insertion for hemodialysis. Dial Transplant 1995;24:559–560, 576.

8 Brittinger WD, Strauch M, et al: 16 months experience with the subcutaneously fixed superficial femoral artery for chronic haemodialysis. Proc Eur Dial Transplant Assoc 1970; 7:408–412.

9 Murotani N, Haruguchi H: Method of superficialized artery access – indication, procedure and management; in: Vascular Access – Actual Review of Construction, Management and Reconstruction (in Japanese). Tokyo, Chyugaiigaku-sha, 2007, pp 49–57.

10 Agishi T, Haruguchi H: Current status of vascular access for chronic hemodialysis patients (in Japanese). Clin Dial 2001;16:1447–1452.

11 Current status of dialysis therapy in Japan (as of December 31, 2008) (in Japanese). Jpn Soc Dial Ther 2010;43:1–35.

12 Murotani N, Hori S, Matsuda Y, Shimada T, Kouno Y, Asano K: Indication of superficialized artery access (in Japanese). Jin to Touseki 2003, pp 7–9.

13 Hamada H, Takada J, Tsuji Y, Katsuki Y, Itami Y, Ohira S: Prognosis of superficialized artery access (in Japanese). Kidney Dial 2003, pp 14–17.

14 Krönung G: Plastic deformation of Cimino fistula by repeated puncture. Dial Transplant 1984;13:635–638.



Kunihiro Hayakawa, MD
Satsukinomori Clinic
1665-2 Nakase, Hamakita-ku, Hamamatsu
Shizuoka-ken (Japan)
E-Mail hayakawa@1985.jukuin.keio.ac.jp

# Author Index

# Subject Index